The Smallest Girl in the Smallest Grade

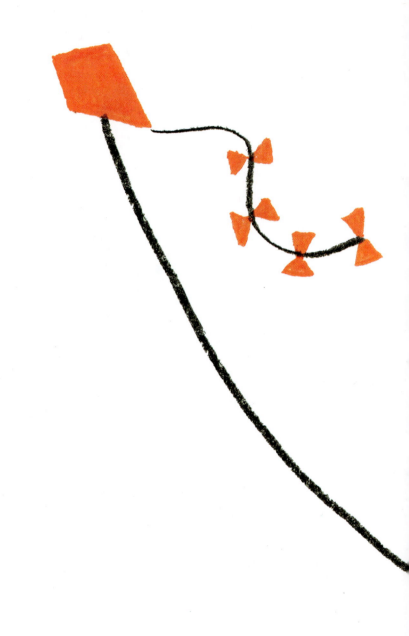
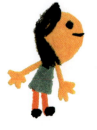

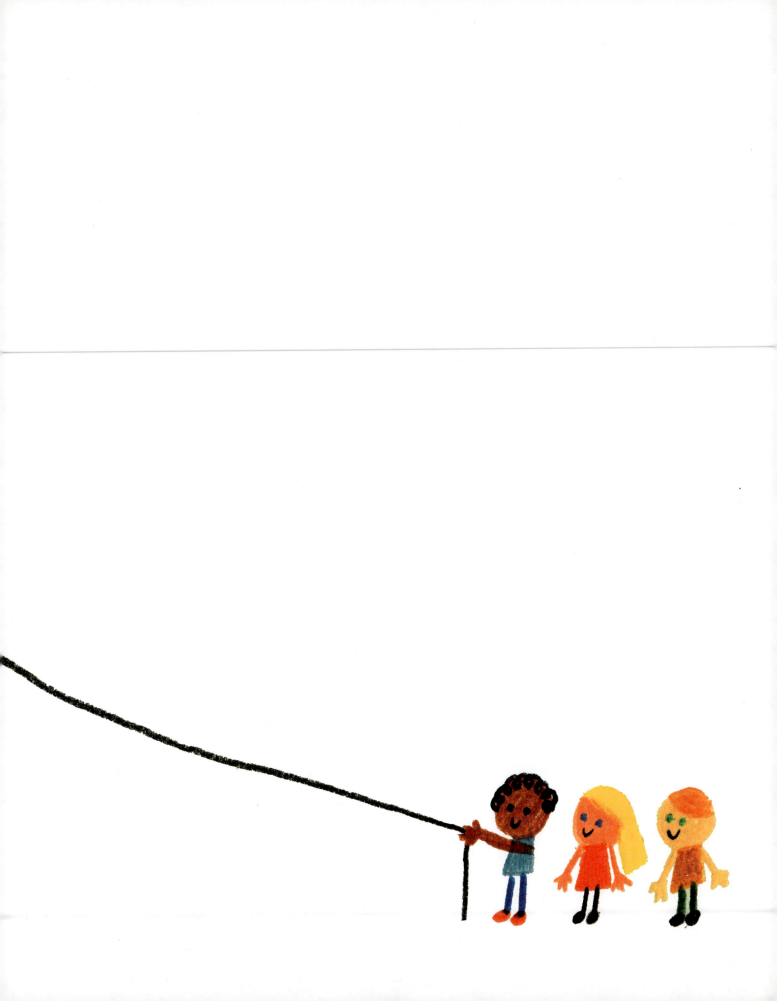

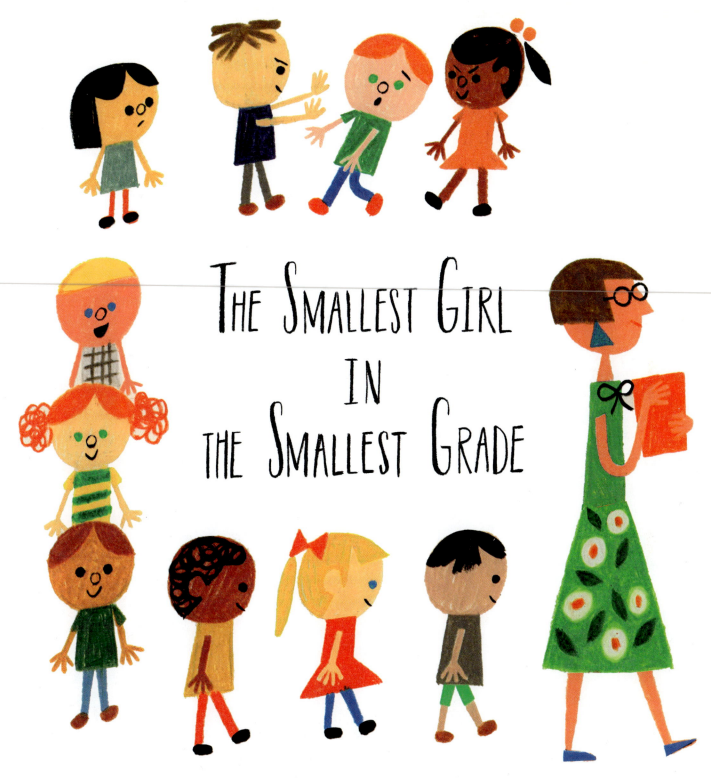

The Smallest Girl in the Smallest Grade

written by
JUSTIN ROBERTS

illustrated by
CHRISTIAN ROBINSON

SCHOLASTIC INC.

Hardly anyone noticed young Sally McCabe.

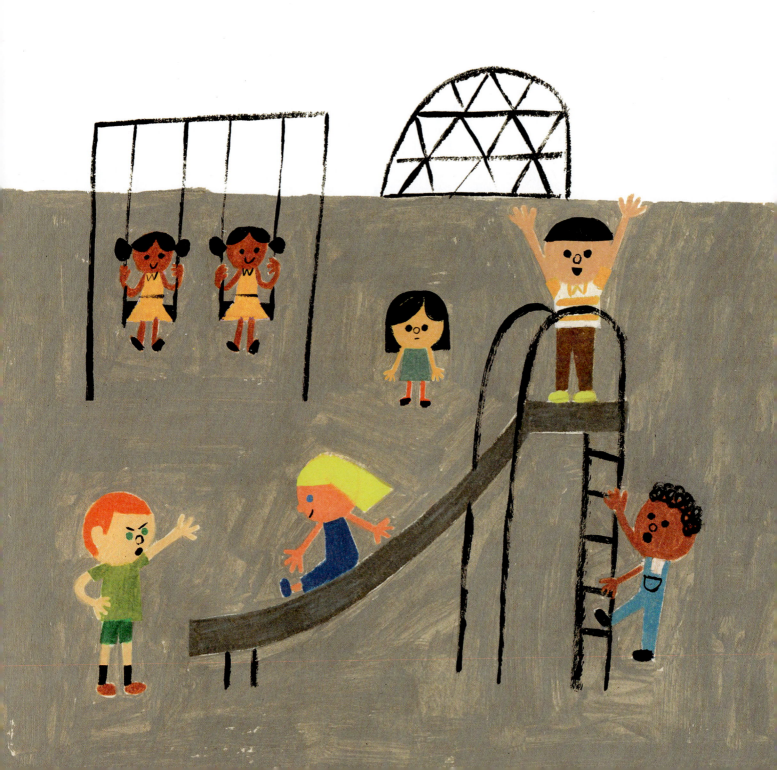

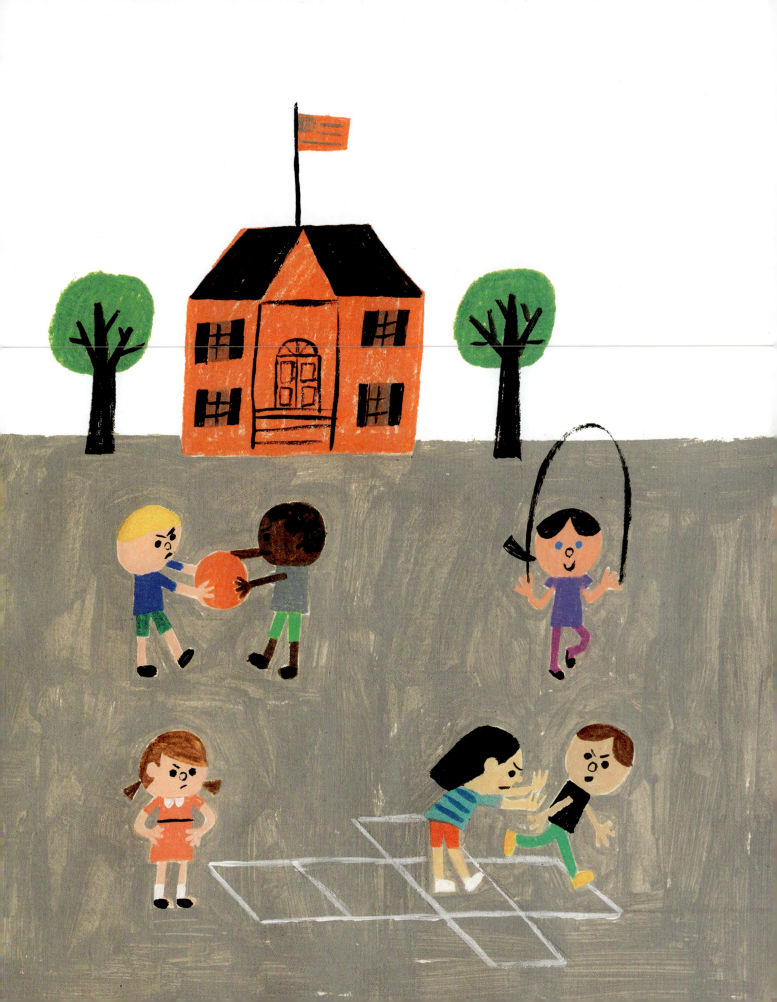

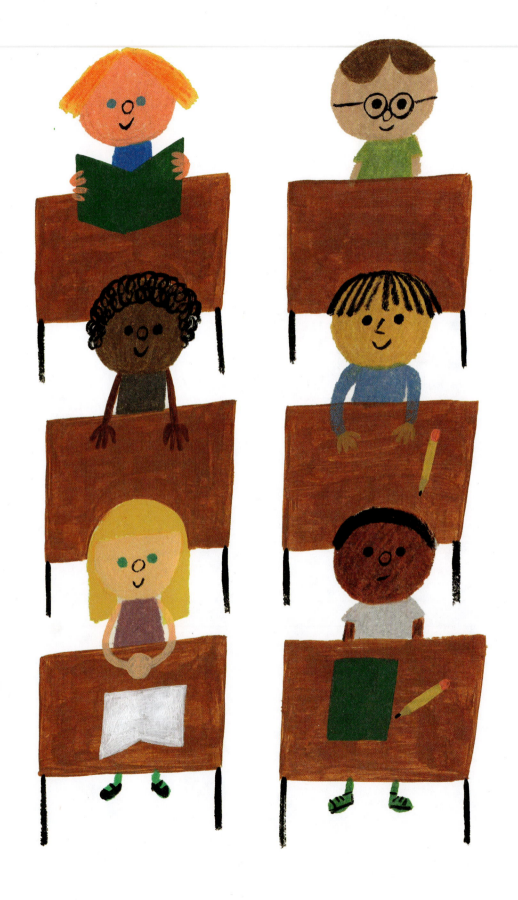

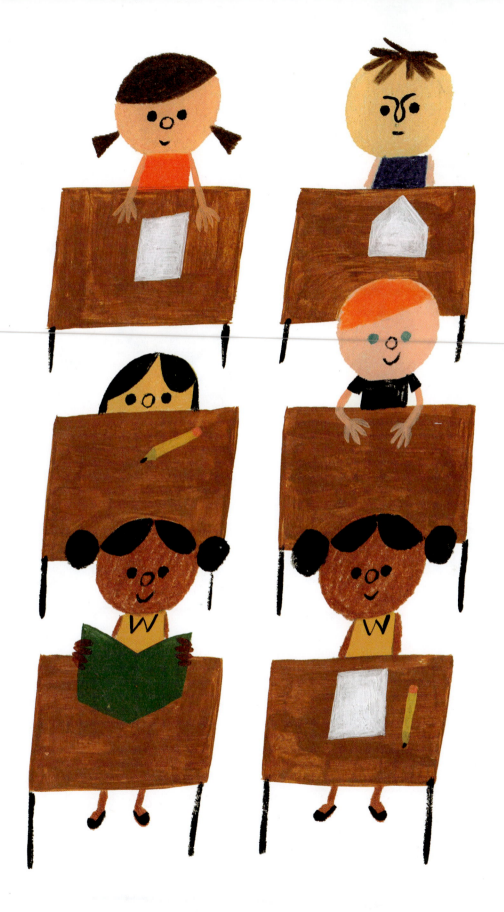

She was the smallest girl in the smallest grade.

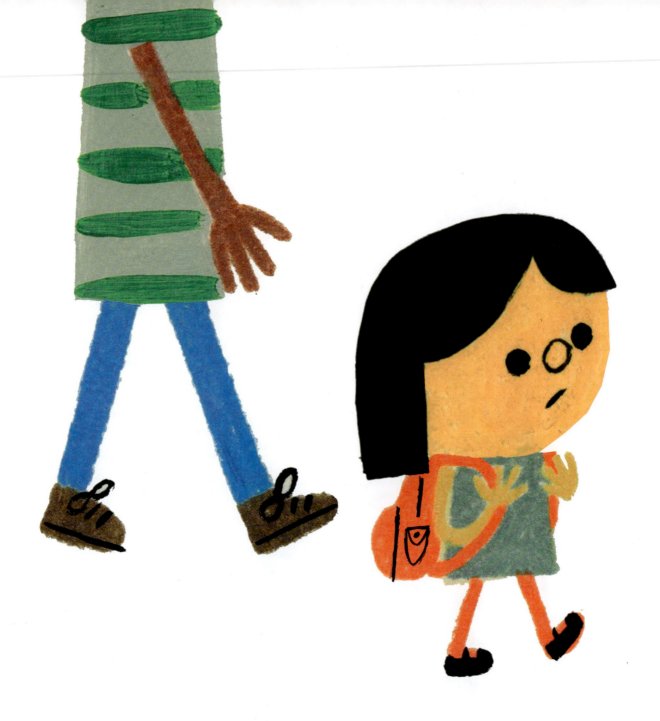

Sure, her name could be heard in the daily roll call,
and she marched with her books down the same school hall.
But hardly anyone noticed young Sally McCabe.

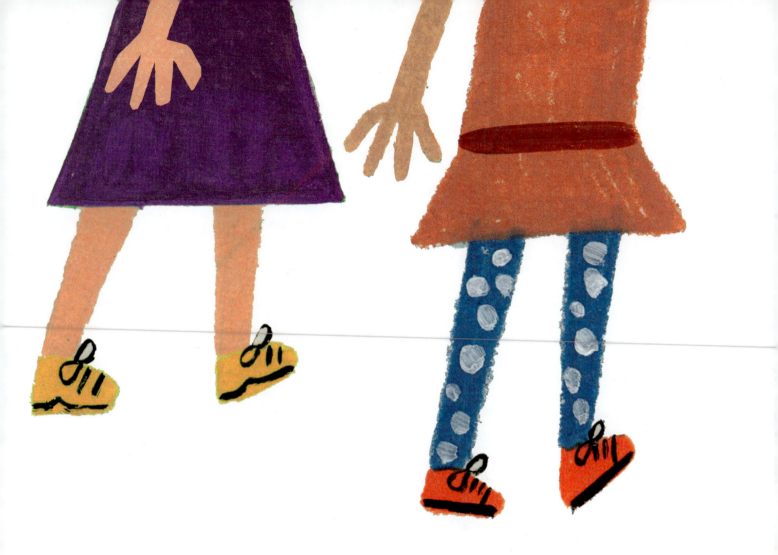

And they certainly didn't know, or at least didn't mention,
that Sally was paying super extra special attention.

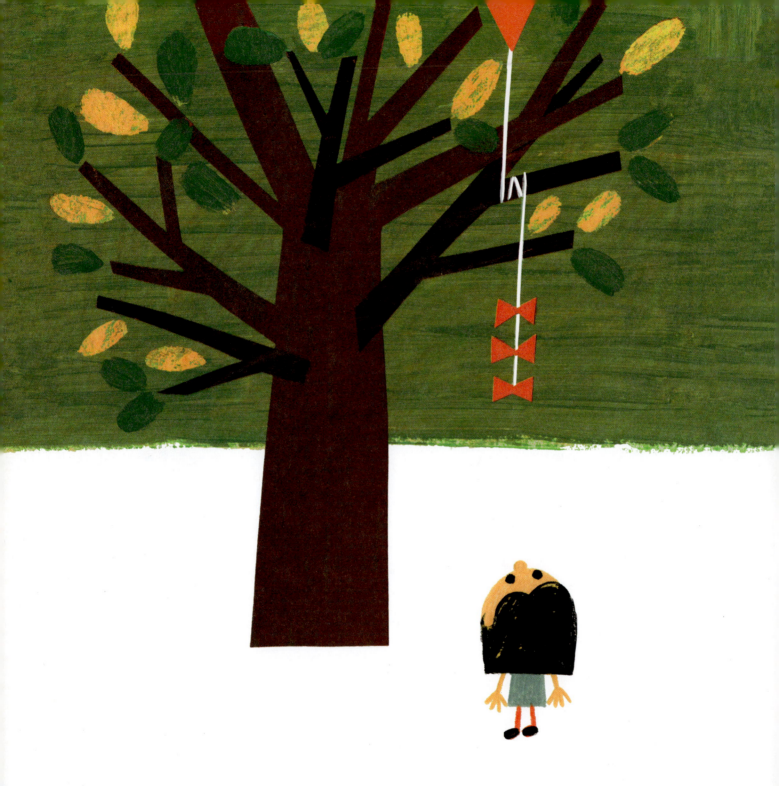

To the abandoned kite with the tangled string.
To the twenty-seven keys on the janitor's ring.

To the leaves as they turned green to gold in the fall.
To the time Tommy Torino was tripped in the hall.

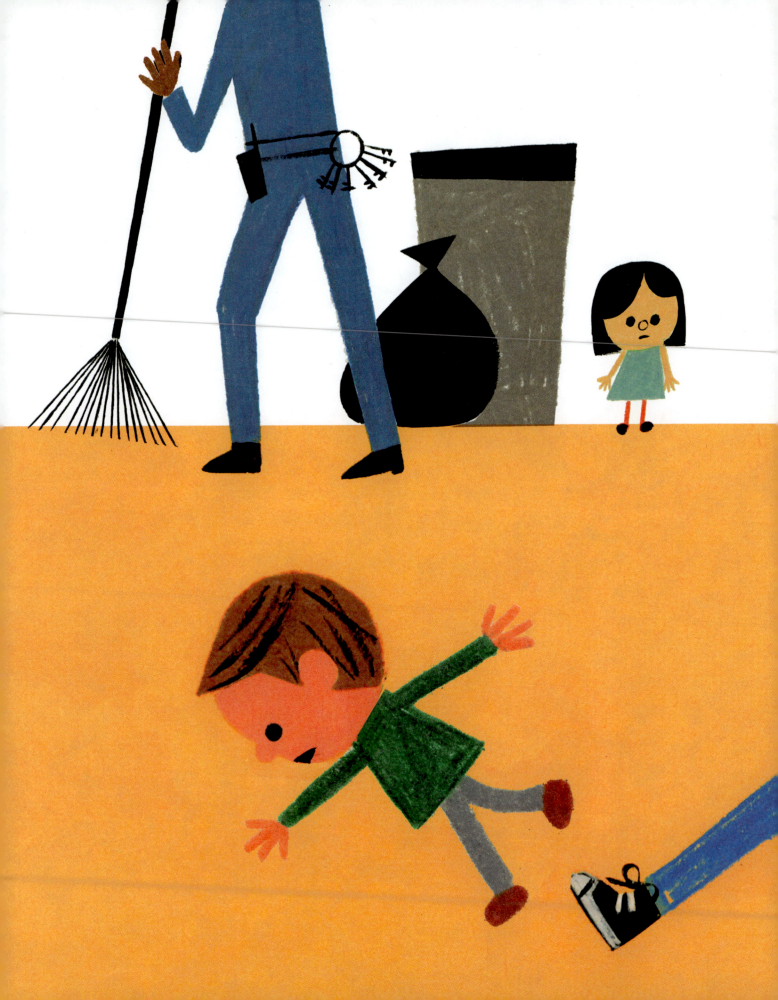

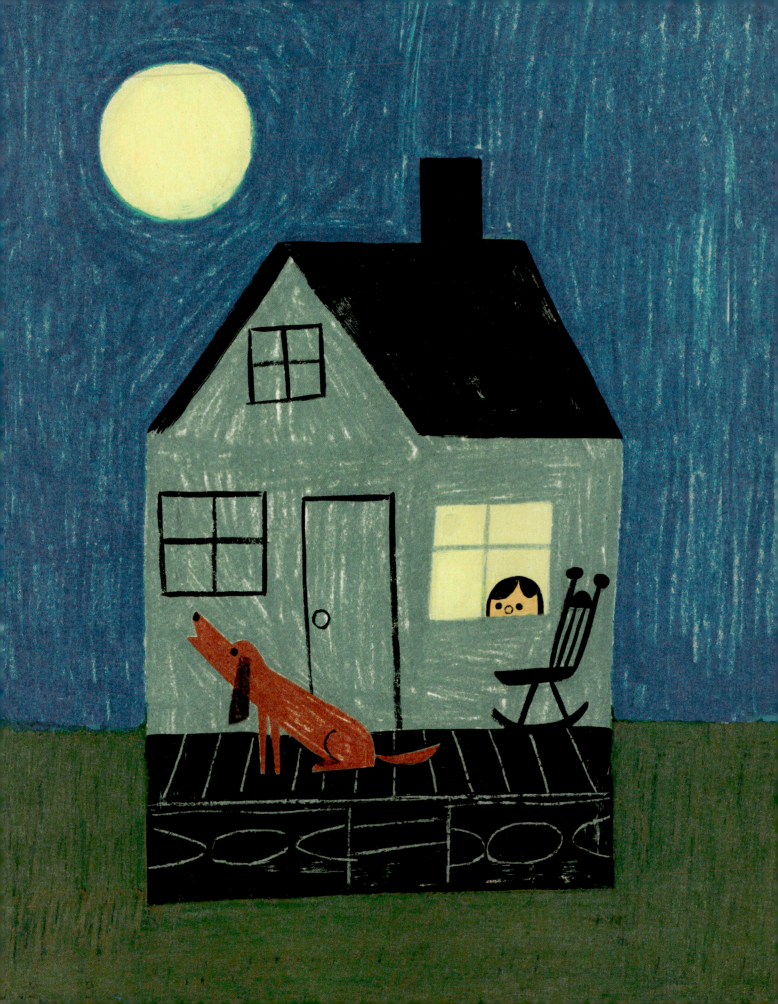

She watched as the wildflowers tipped toward the light,
and heard the howl of a hound dog late one night.

She was there when the stray cats who normally fought
conducted a meeting in the church parking lot.

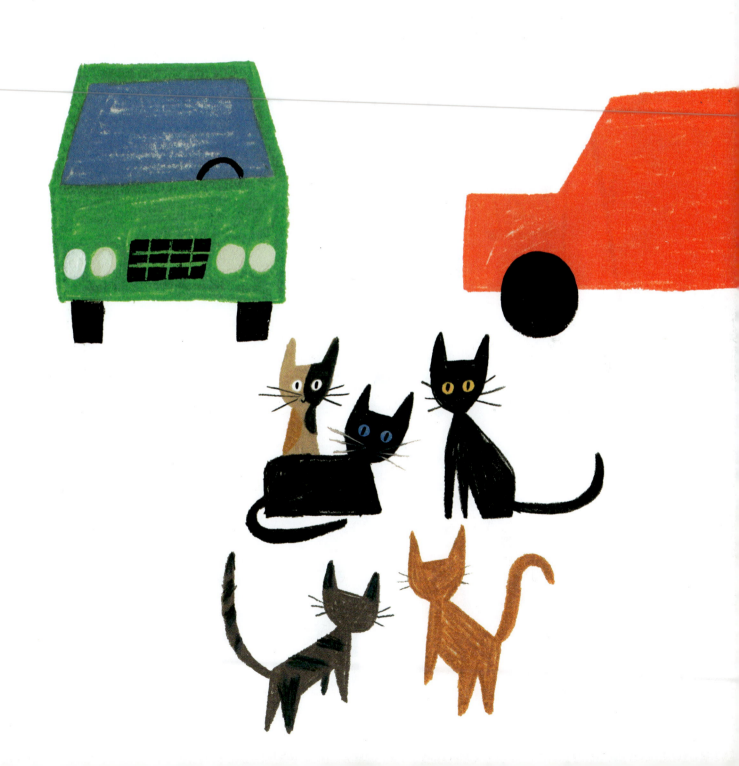

She saw Kevin McKuen get pushed off a slide—
and the oncoming tears that he wanted to hide.

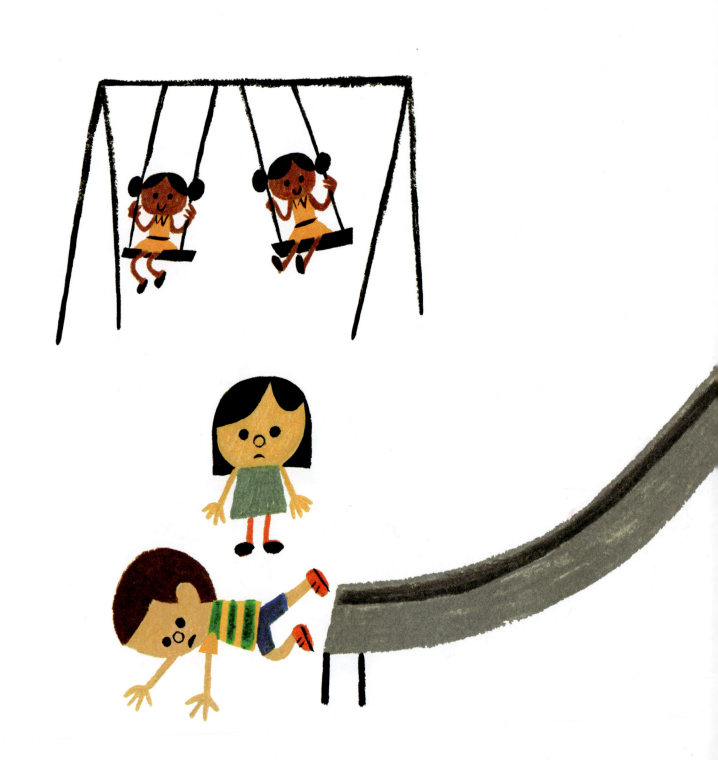

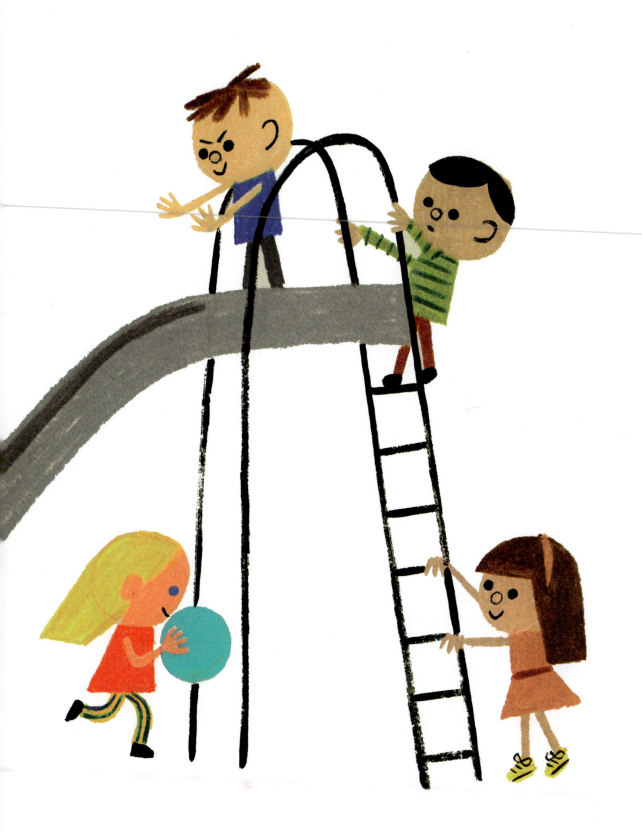

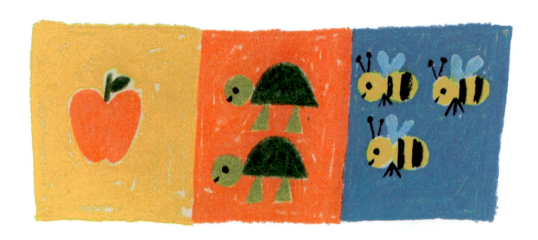

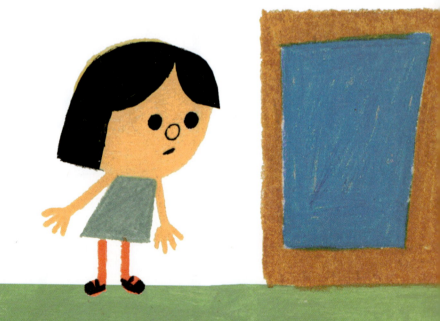

And she'll never forget that Parent-Teacher Day
when Billy's much larger father suddenly dragged him away.

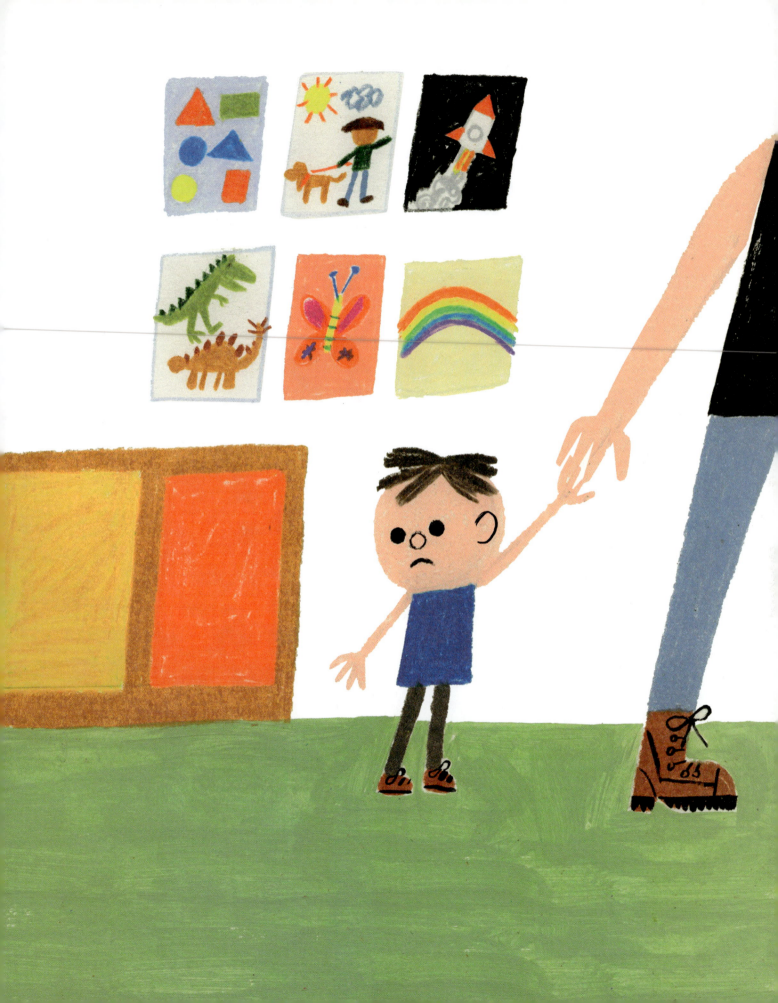

But through all the mean words and all the cold stares,
no one even noticed that Sally was there.
And they certainly didn't know, or at least didn't mention,
that Sally was paying super extra special attention.

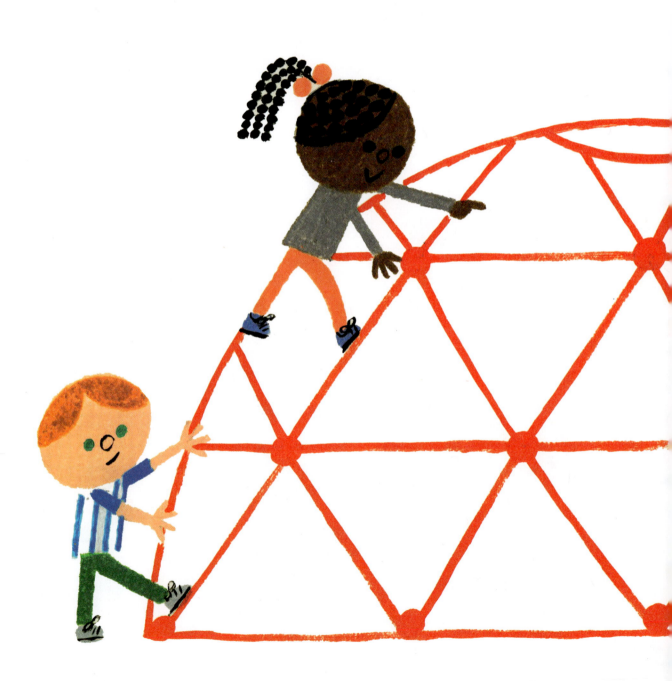

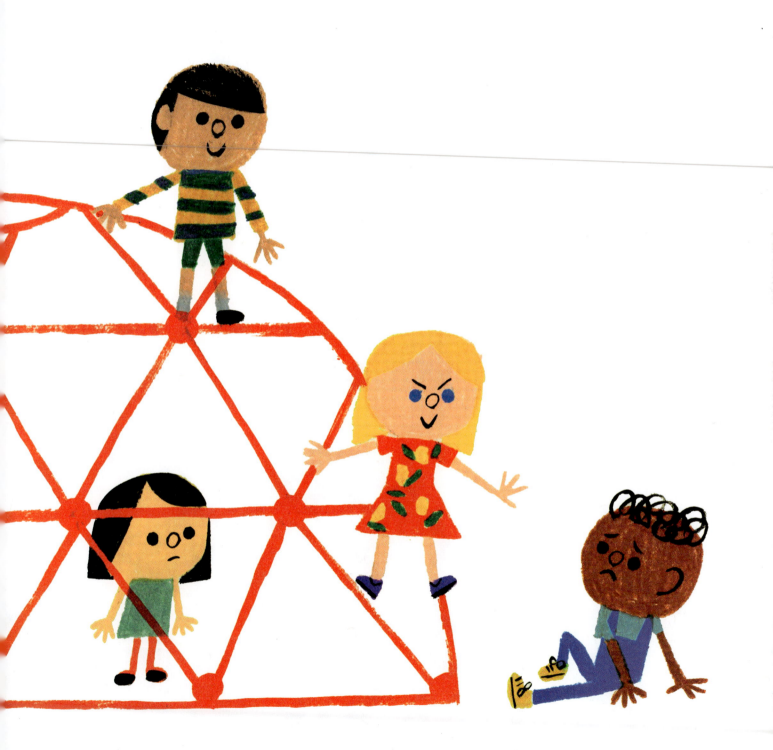

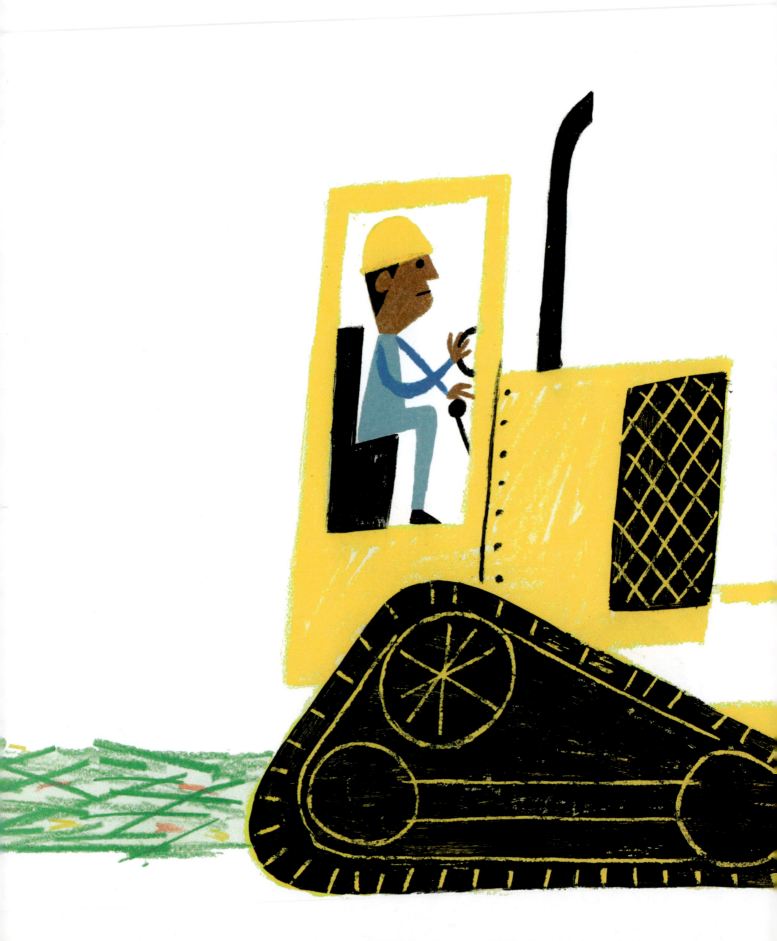

She'd seen how a whisper could make someone cower
like a bulldozer crushing through fields of wildflowers.
And it kept piling up, this discarded debris,
those beautiful kites tangled in trees.

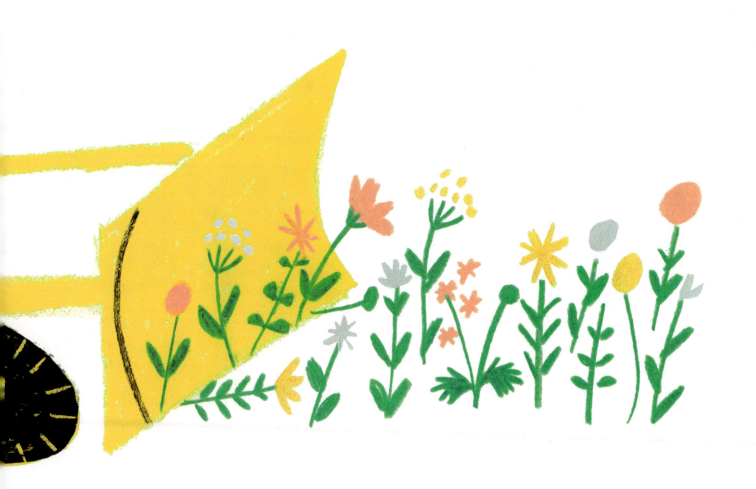

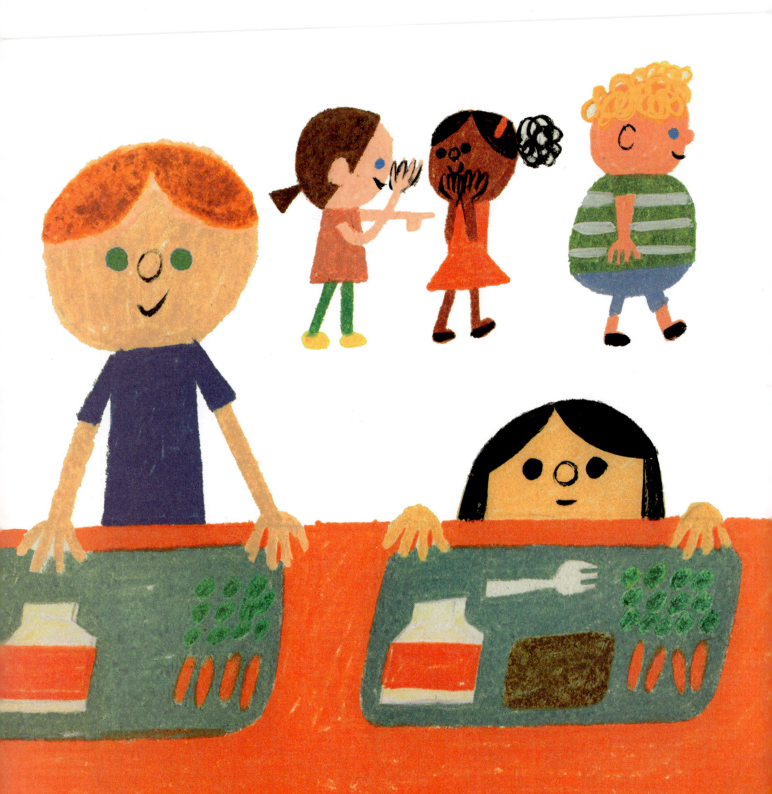

So on February third at eleven twenty-nine,
Sally stepped straight out of the lunchroom line.

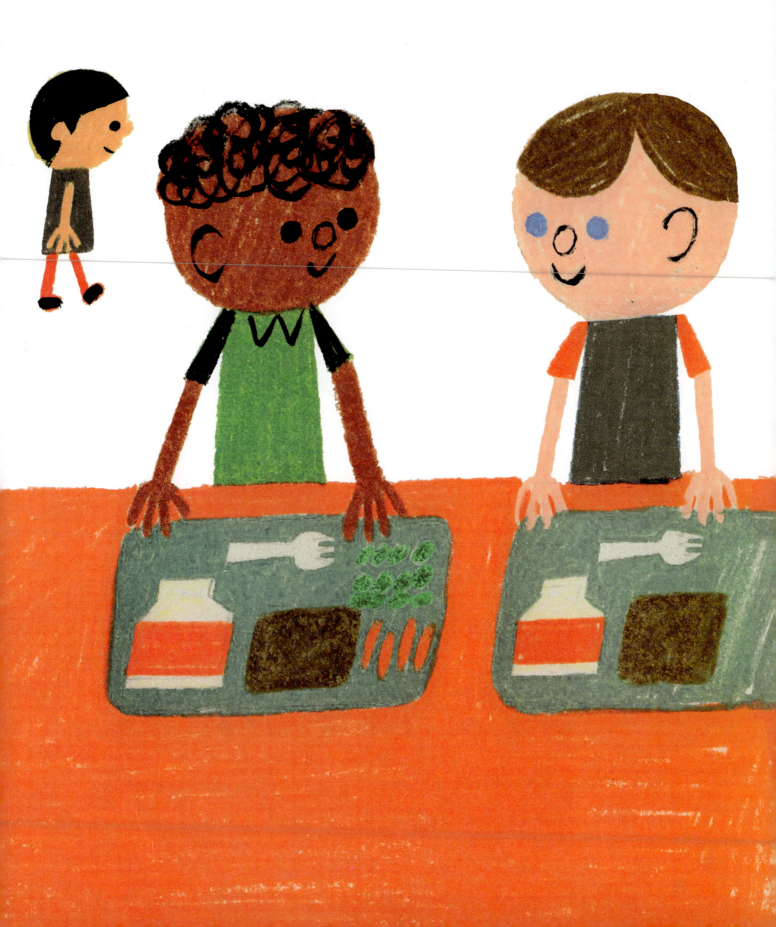

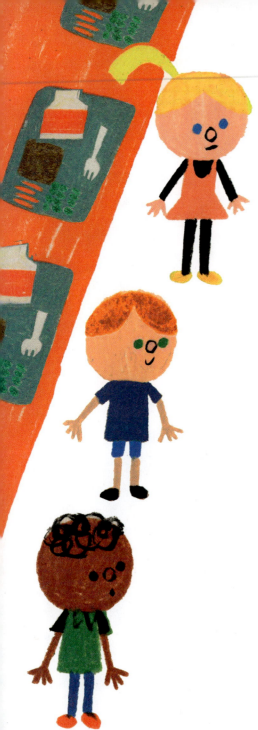

She said, "I'm tired of seeing this terrible stuff.
Stop hurting each other! This is enough!"

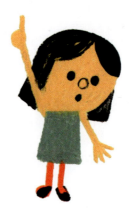

Now, a few laughed out loud or didn't care
that there was some girl with her hand in the air.

But then something super extra special happened that day
as Howard O'Henry suddenly set down his tray.

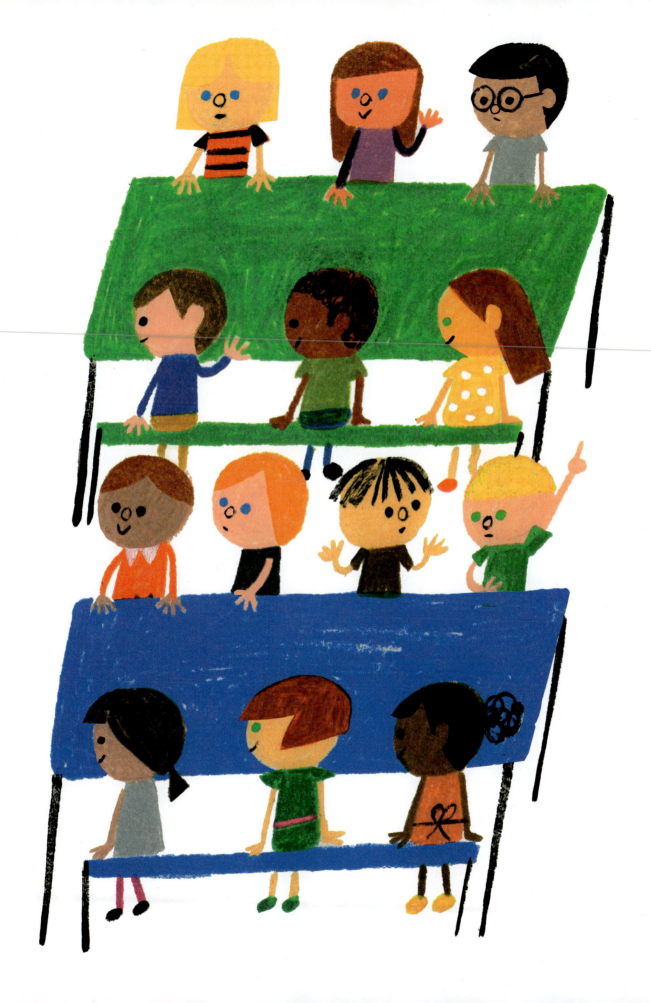

Like waves rolling in, one after another—
first Molly rose up, then Michael's twin brother.
It was Tyrone and Terence, then Amanda and Paul,
who pushed out their chairs and stretched their arms tall.

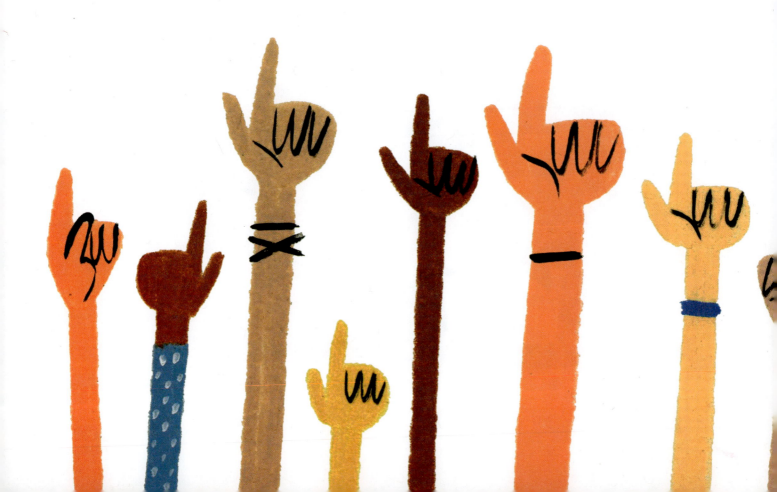

From the friendly lunch lady with the dishes she carted,
to that new third-grade teacher who had only recently started.
Yes, everyone there, even Principal Claire,
had joined little Sally with their fingers in the air.

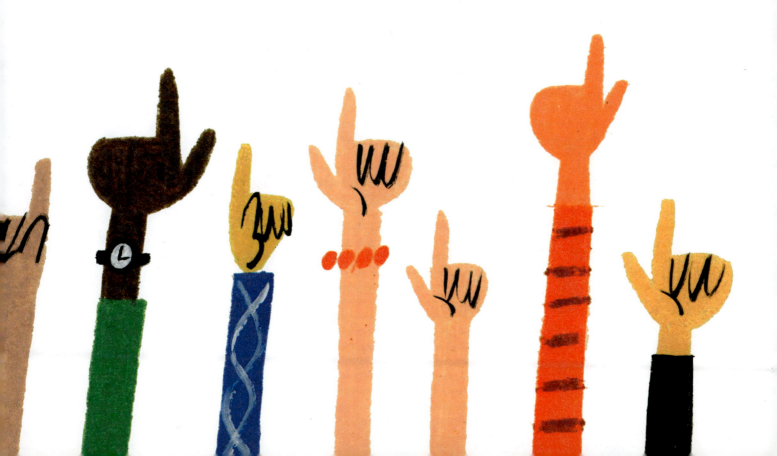

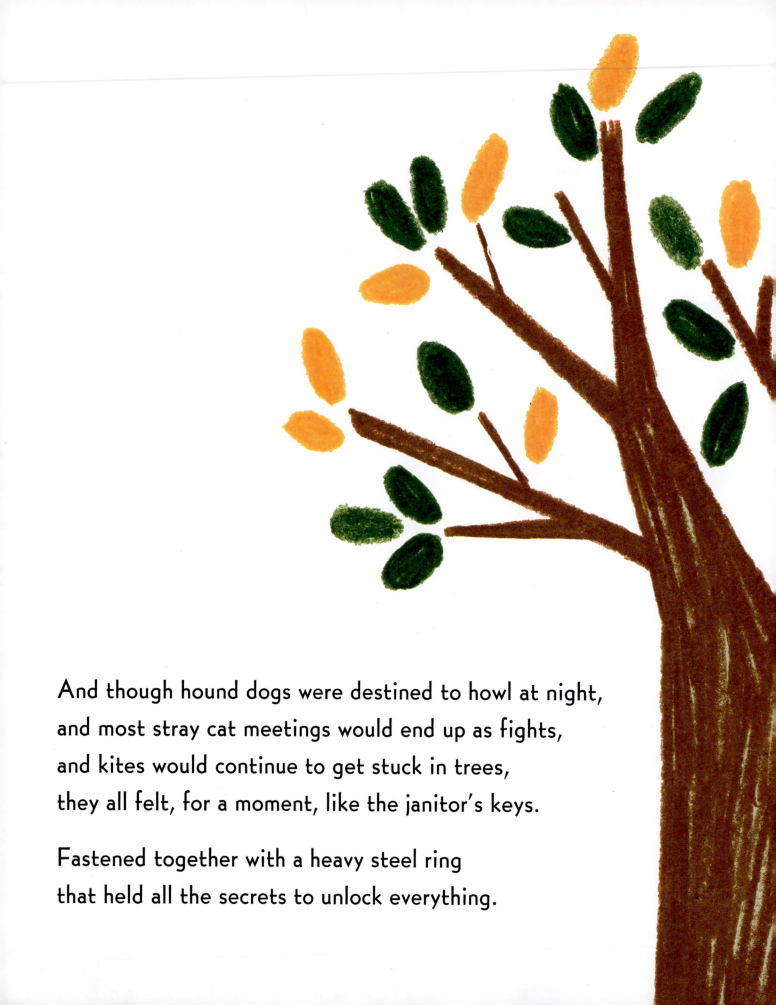

And though hound dogs were destined to howl at night,
and most stray cat meetings would end up as fights,
and kites would continue to get stuck in trees,
they all felt, for a moment, like the janitor's keys.

Fastened together with a heavy steel ring
that held all the secrets to unlock everything.

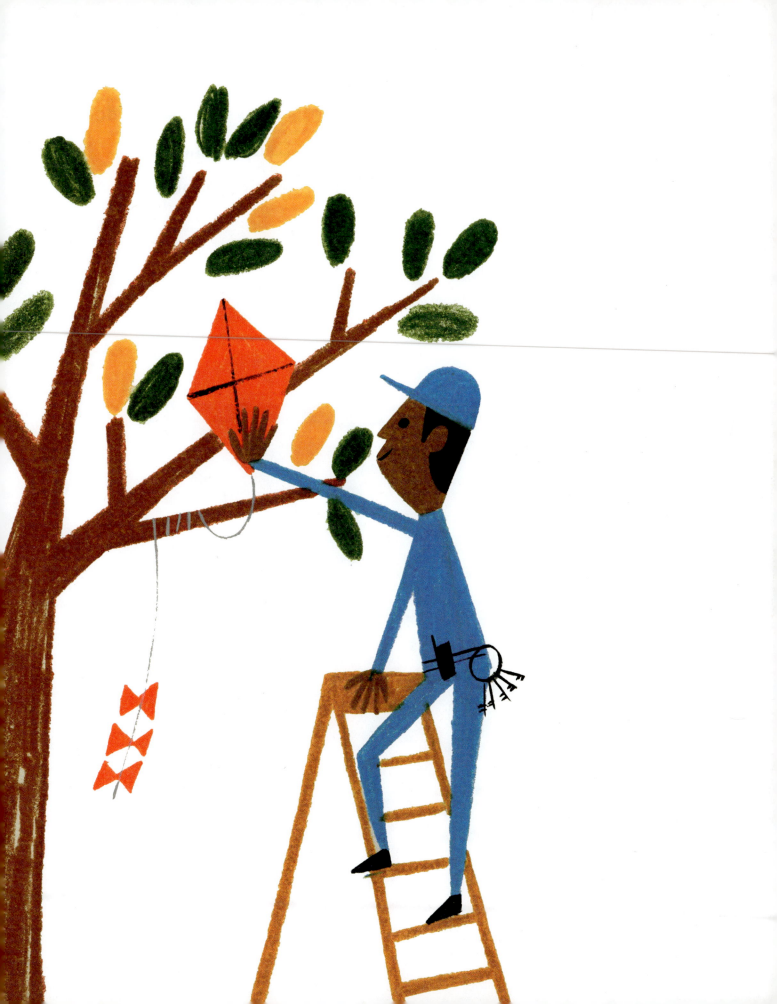

As the world returned to the way that it was,
Sally noticed the difference, as she usually does,
when Billy paused briefly to open the door
for Mrs. O'Connell and seventeen more.

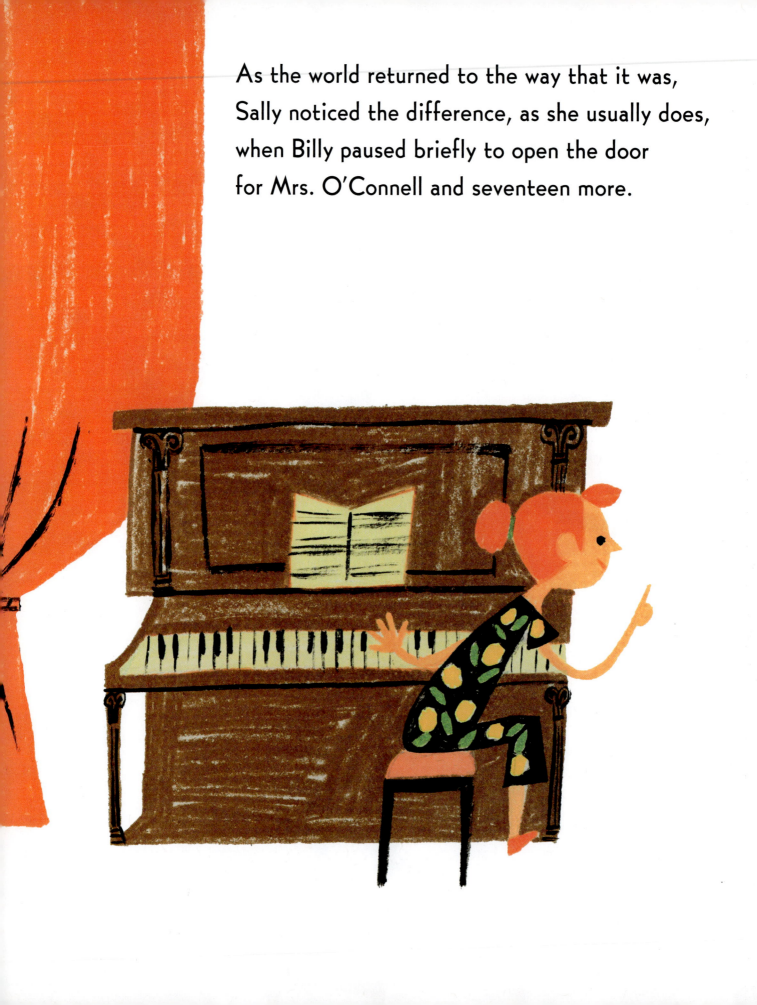

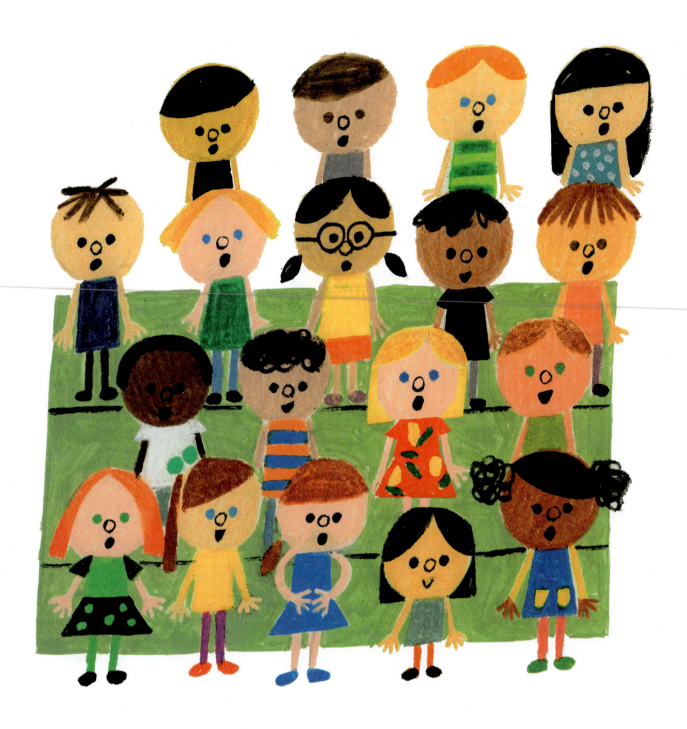

Or when Molly scooched over to make some space
on the choral riser for Ellen and Grace.
These moments that often get taken for granted—
a wildflower appearing that no one had planted.

The swings soon resumed their rhythm and sway,
and day turned to night and night turned to day.

People remembered and would quite often mention
that Sally had been paying super extra special attention.
And how the world could transform and a change could be made
by the smallest girl in the smallest grade.

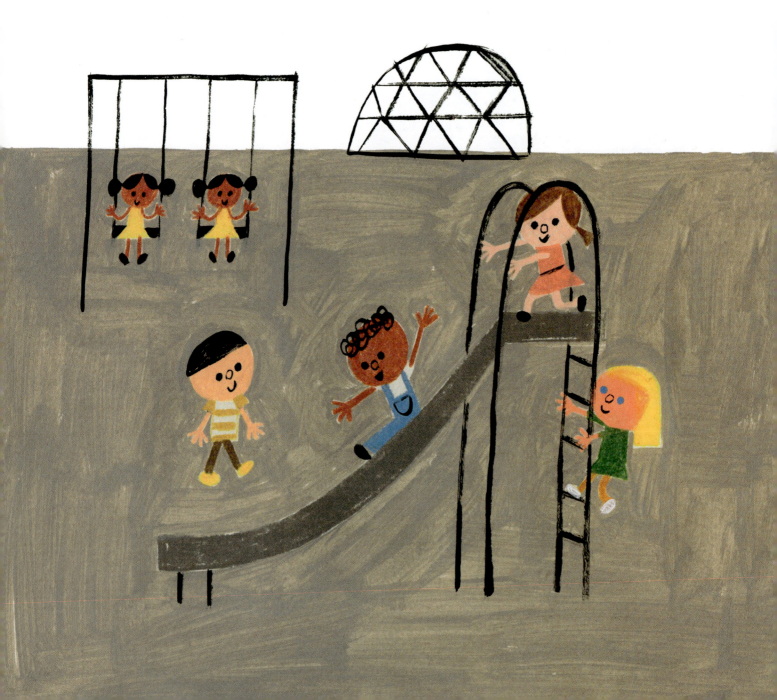

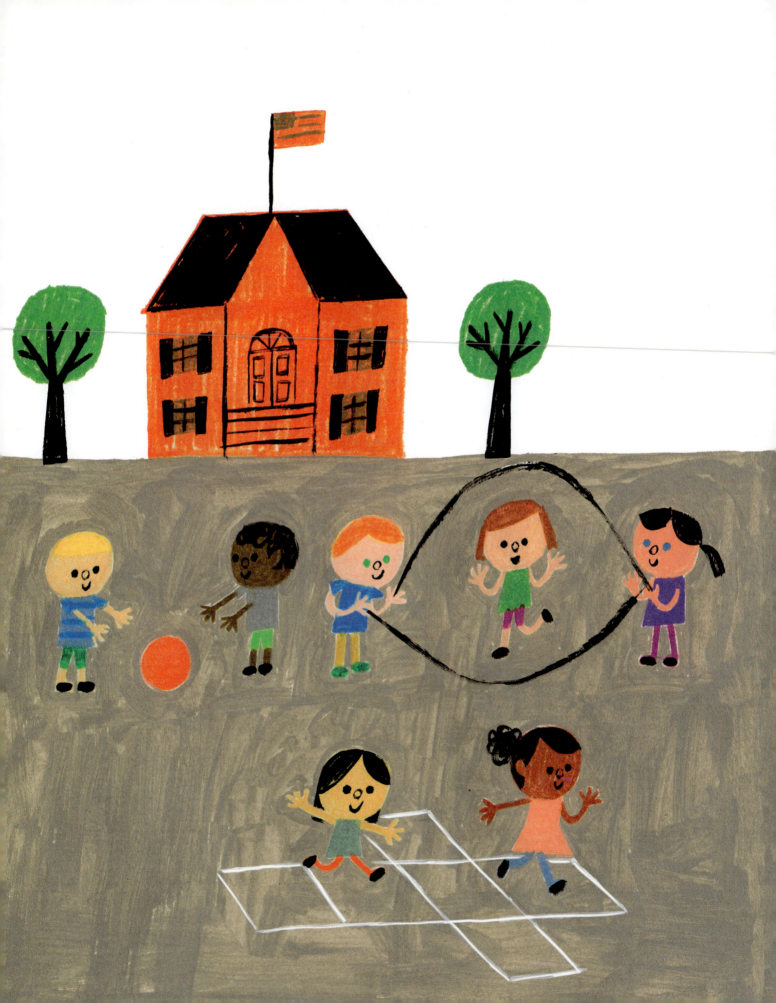

To all those paying
super extra special attention.
—J.R.

To Yvonne.
Thank you for standing up for me.
—C.R.

ISBN 978-1-338-14934-0

12 11 10 9 8 7 6 5 4 3 2 1   16 17 18 19 20 21

Printed in the U.S.A.   40

This edition first printing, September 2016

Design by Ryan Thomann
Text set in Bernhard Gothic
The art for this book was done in colored pencil.

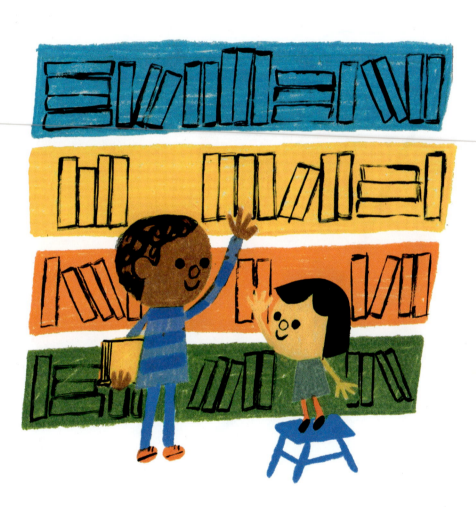

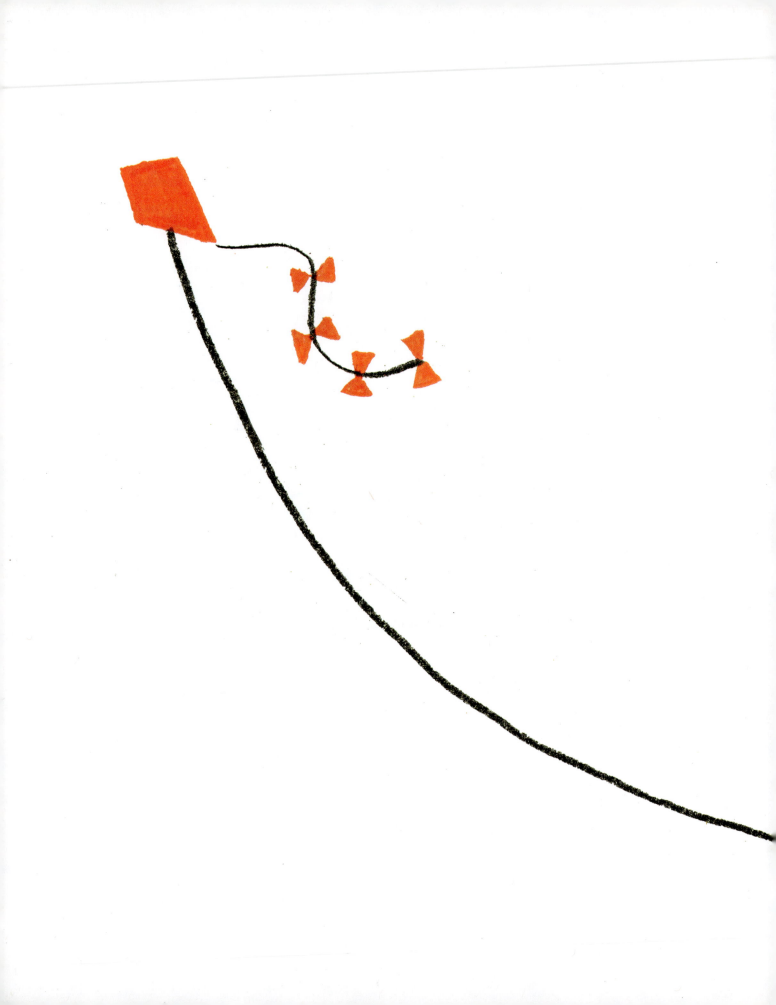

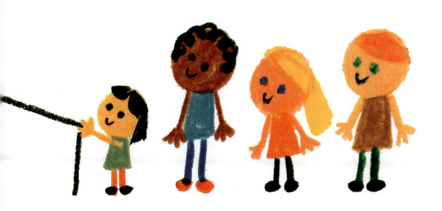

Table of contents (front)

Have more questions about growing a little human?

Mayo Clinic Guide to a Healthy Pregnancy has lots of answers.

Mayo Clinic Guide to a Healthy Pregnancy provides additional information for all parents-to-be. It's a comprehensive resource for every stage of pregnancy and a reference manual you can trust. In this book, you'll find extensive guidance and practical tips, including:

· Evidence-based medical advice for parents from a world-class team of doctors and care providers

· Information on pregnancy planning and fertility

· Weekly updates on baby's growth and development

· Monthly explanations of changes for mom

· Guidance on nutrition, exercise and weight gain

· Tips for working, traveling and managing parenthood

· Reliable information on recent trends and technologies in pregnancy and postpartum care

· Answers to difficult or embarrassing questions

Order Mayo Clinic books and newsletters online at
Marketplace.MayoClinic.com

When you purchase books from Mayo Clinic Press, you help support Mayo Clinic programs, including medical education and research.

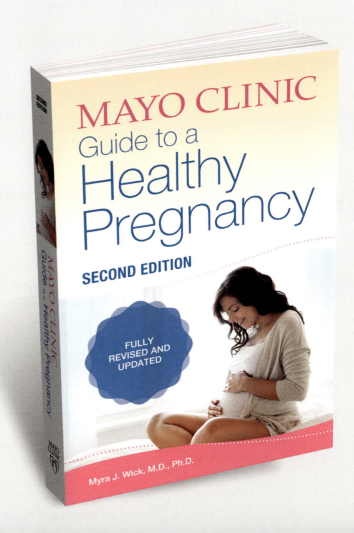

Table of contents (back)

Parenthood is an adventure.
Find guidance from Mayo Clinic experts.

Mayo Clinic Guide to Your Baby's First Years is an
essential resource for new or experienced parents. This second
edition extends practical guidance on caring for your child from
birth to age 3. Inside you'll find evidence-based advice on issues
such as eating and nutrition, healthy sleep habits, fussiness and
tantrums, and bonding with your child. Also included are monthly
growth and development updates, tips for juggling work and family,
and much more.

Mayo Clinic Guide to Raising a Healthy Child offers a
trusted guide to parenting your child through the preschool and
early school-age years. It provides answers to dilemmas such as
feeding a picky eater, resolving sleep problems, addressing bullying,
treating common injuries and illnesses, and coping with complex
health care needs. You'll also find expert insights on shaping your
child's behavior in a positive way, increasing your child's resilience
and cultivating a warm, supportive environment for your family.

When you purchase books from Mayo Clinic Press, you help support
Mayo Clinic programs, including medical education and research.

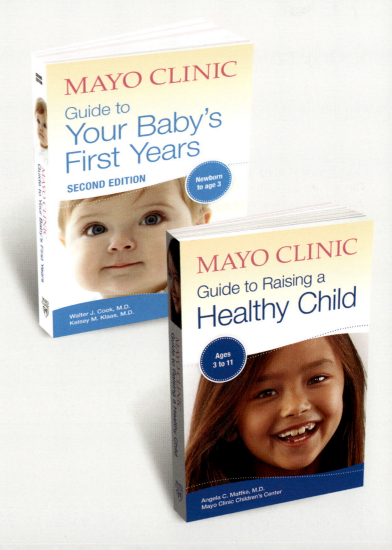

#3

Congratulations!

"Pregnant and birthing mothers are elemental forces, in the same sense that gravity, thunderstorms, earthquakes and hurricanes are elemental forces. In order to understand the laws of their energy flow, you have to love and respect them for their magnificence at the same time that you study them with the accuracy of a true scientist."

—Ina May Gaskin

Huge, heartfelt congrats as you anticipate a baby joining your family! The journey of pregnancy and childbirth is like no other. Each birth is a truly unique experience — one that can shape parenthood, build confidence, and leave a lasting impression on mother, baby and family.

We share in your goal of giving your baby the very best start in life. A positive birth experience stems from a combination of education, comfort techniques and an understanding of options. This book offers all of those, backed by research and the expertise of doctors, midwives, nurses and doulas.

Each page offers a concise run-down of key topics to help you enter labor with confidence. The information here aims to help you learn the wide range of what's normal during pregnancy, labor and childbirth, so that you can stay at ease when you recognize something as part of the process. This book also explores what's possible, so you know the potential of this amazing adventure.

Everyone brings unique histories, beliefs and traditions to childbirth. Whatever your hopes and plans for your birth, we hope that this book can help lead you to a safe, healthy and joyous delivery.

Please note: The FRONT pages consist of the most important information to equip you for a positive childbirth experience. Soak up that knowledge first. Then, flip the book around to the BACK pages for more ah-ha moments and empowerment for pregnancy, labor and beyond. The book's lay-flat binding means that you can take it in while eating breakfast, riding a stationary bike or lounging in bed.

Health and happiness to you and yours!

Julie and Kerry

Image credits

The individuals pictured are models, and the photos are used for illustrative purposes only. There is no correlation between the individuals portrayed and the subjects being discussed.

All photographs and illustrations are copyright of MFMER, except for the following:

#4

About us

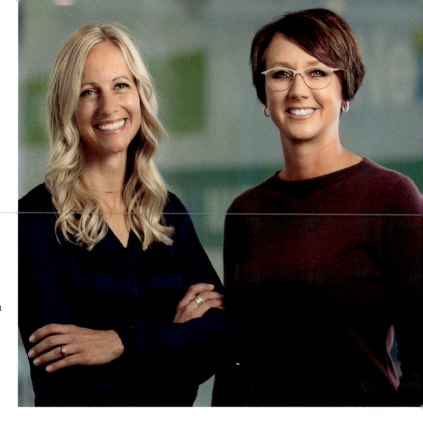

Julie Lamppa (*right*), APRN, Certified Nurse-Midwife (CNM) at Mayo Clinic, Rochester, Minn., and mother of two

Julie's career has been dedicated to caring for pregnant and laboring women. She was a labor and delivery nurse for 15 years before earning a master's degree in midwifery in 2009. In addition to working as a midwife, she is a clinical instructor in the Department of Obstetrics and Gynecology at the Mayo Clinic College of Medicine and Science and a contributing editor of *Mayo Clinic Guide to a Healthy Pregnancy*. From extensive experience with low- and higher-risk pregnancies, Julie knows things don't always go as planned. She believes that helping women be well informed can lead to better birth experiences in any situation.

Kerry Schwalbach, Certified Labor Doula, Certified Postpartum Doula and mama of three

Kerry began training as a doula through DONA International in 2008. Early on, she wondered why some of the concepts and tips she learned for supporting women in labor weren't on billboards for pregnant women everywhere. After putting her expertise to use with her own second and third births, she was determined to help spread such empowering information. Kerry's 20+ years in the wellness field include roles as a health educator, Pilates instructor, and consultant for the development of prenatal media and a family wellness curriculum. She sees pregnancy as an opportunity for a woman to focus on her health, gaining tools and tricks she can continue to use as her family grows.

MAYO CLINIC

Editorial Director
Paula M. Marlow Limbeck

Senior Editor
Karen R. Wallevand

Managing Editor
Anna L. Cavallo

Senior Product Manager
Daniel J. Harke

Art Director
Stewart J. Koski

Production
Darren L. Wendt

Editorial Research Librarians
Abbie Y. Brown, Edward (Eddy) S. Morrow Jr., Erika A. Riggin, Katherine (Katie) J. Warner

Copy Editors
Miranda M. Attlesey, Alison K. Baker, Nancy J. Jacoby, Julie M. Maas

Contributors
Ying Ying (Christina) Chen, M.D.; Rebekah L. Huppert, R.N., I.B.C.L.C.; Denise M. Millstine, M.D.; Liz Naylor, C.D. (DONA), I.B.C.L.C.; Kristi M. Urban, R.N.; Angela C. Thompson, M.D., M.P.H.; Myra J. Wick, M.D., Ph.D.

Special thanks to: Eleena, Nathan and Sydney Koep; Erin, John and Doca Pepelnjak; Kamber, Steven and McKinley Schneider; Kerry, John and Sam Schwalbach

Published by Mayo Clinic Press

© 2021 Mayo Foundation for Medical Education and Research (MFMER)

The information in this book is true and complete to the best of our knowledge. This book is intended only as an informative guide for those wishing to learn more about health issues. It is not intended to replace, countermand or conflict with advice given to you by your own physician. The ultimate decision concerning your care should be made between you and your doctor. Information in this book is offered with no guarantees. The authors and publisher disclaim all liability in connection with the use of this book.

For bulk sales to employers, member groups and health-related companies, contact Mayo Clinic, 200 First St. SW, Rochester, MN 55905, or send an email to *SpecialSalesMayoBooks@mayo.edu*.

ISBN 978-1-893005-64-8

Library of Congress Control Number: 2020949968

Printed in the United States of America

#5

Food for thought

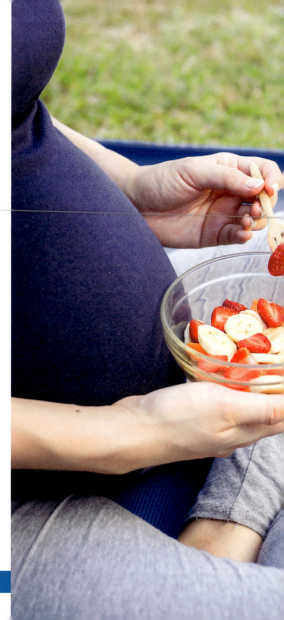

Pregnancy is a vital time for you and your growing baby. Prenatal nutrition can have a profound long-term effect on baby's health. Think of baby as a motivating personal trainer, keeping you on track — feeling energized, fit and strong. (If morning sickness is a struggle, talk with your medical provider.)

- EAT A WELL-BALANCED DIET, including adequate protein, healthy fats, limited sugar, and lots of vegetables and fruits.
- TELL YOUR FRIENDS! FOLATE is vitamin B-9, and it helps prevent serious problems with a baby's brain and spinal cord (neural tube defects). This means ALL women who could become pregnant should get adequate amounts of this vitamin — 400 to 800 micrograms (mcg) daily. Great natural sources include leafy greens, asparagus, broccoli, beans, peas, lentils, citrus fruits, beets, eggs, avocados, Brussels sprouts, bananas, nuts and seeds. FOLIC ACID is the synthetic form of folate, found in vitamins and fortified foods. Another form that's sometimes found in vitamins is L-METHYLFOLATE.
- DRINK LOTS OF WATER (about 64 ounces a day) instead of sugary drinks, for overall hydration without excess calories.
- TAKE A PRENATAL VITAMIN WITH IRON to help baby grow strong and to avoid anemia as your blood volume increases. During pregnancy, aim to get 27 milligrams (mg) of iron daily. Most pregnant women will need added iron in their diet — through a vitamin or supplement and iron-rich foods. Iron from animal sources is most easily absorbed, but dried beans and peas are great plant options. Other supplements to consider include vitamin D-3, omega-3 fatty acids, probiotics and calcium.

#108

WHERE TO LOOK FOR MORE DISCUSSION, RESEARCH AND SUPPORT

ONLINE

American Academy of Pediatrics
www.aap.org
The latest news and research, helpful tips, and more

American College of Nurse-Midwives
www.midwife.org
Information and essential facts about midwives

American College of Obstetricians and Gynecologists
www.acog.org/patients
Fact sheets, videos and many FAQs from childbirth experts

DONA International
www.dona.org
Information about doulas from a leading international professional organization, as well as a directory to find a doula

La Leche League International
www.llli.org
Supportive information and resources on breastfeeding

Lamaze International
www.lamaze.org
Information on pregnancy, labor and classes (in person or online)

Mayo Clinic
www.mayoclinic.org
Mayo Clinic's online information portal, including many resources on pregnancy

BOOKS

Gaskin IM. *Ina May's Guide to Childbirth*. Bantam Books Trade Paperbacks; 2019. An enduring guide to natural childbirth from a leading midwife.

Simkin P. *The Birth Partner: A Complete Guide to Childbirth for Dads, Doulas, and Other Labor Companions*. 5th ed. Harvard Common Press; 2018. An iconic handbook from a doula and physical therapist with a specialty in childbirth education.

SUPPORTING RESEARCH CITED FOR KEY IDEAS

American College of Obstetricians and Gynecologists. Committee Opinion No. 766: Approaches to limit intervention during labor and birth. Obstetrics & Gynecology. 2019; doi:10.1097/AOG.0000000000003074.

Bohren MA, et al. Continuous support for women during childbirth. Cochrane Database of Systematic Reviews. 2017; doi: 10.1002/14651858.CD003766.pub6.

Healthy birth practice #6: Keep mother and baby together — it's best for mother, baby, and breastfeeding. Journal of Perinatal Education. 2014; doi:10.1891/1058-1243.23.4.211.

Sharpe EE, et al. Epidural labor analgesia and maternal fever. Clinical Obstetrics and Gynecology. 2017; doi:10.1097/GRF.0000000000000270.

#6

Steer clear

BEST TO AVOID:
- Alcohol, CBD, marijuana, tobacco products (including e-cigarettes) and all illicit street drugs.
- Seafood high in mercury, as it could harm baby's developing nervous system. However, you may consume up to 12 ounces (oz.) a week of seafood low in mercury — examples include shrimp, salmon, pollock, cod and canned light tuna. Just don't exceed 6 oz. a week of albacore tuna or tuna steak.
- Foods that could cause listeriosis, a bacterial infection that's 10 times more likely to occur in pregnant women compared with healthy adults. Listeriosis can harm both moms and babies. Steer clear of:
  - Undercooked seafood or meat.
  - Cold hot dogs and processed deli meats. Heat these to steaming or an internal temp of 165 F before eating.
  - Unpasteurized foods, unwashed produce and raw sprouts.
- Excess caffeine (>200 mg in a day).
- High levels of vitamin A. If you take the acne medicine isotretinoin, stop using it before you become pregnant. It can cause birth defects.

ADDITIONAL PRECAUTIONS:
- Always discuss use of medications, vitamins, and natural or herbal products, as well as vaccinations, with your medical provider.
- Wear gloves while doing activities such as gardening or cleaning a litter box, and wash your hands thoroughly afterward.

TO BE EXTRA CAUTIOUS, AVOID OR LIMIT EXPOSURE TO:
- Pesticides, insecticides, paint, varnish and aerosols.
- Harsh household cleaning products.
- Cosmetics and beauty products that may have trace amounts of toxins such as lead, mercury, phthalates and parabens.
- Plastics that aren't BPA-free.
- Wireless technology. Evidence shows no cause for alarm. But if you're nervous about your exposure to electromagnetic energy, try using your cellphone's speaker, and avoid holding your phone and laptop close to your body for long periods.

#107

Love at first sight

An ultrasound image of your baby may look textbook perfect — or barely human! Either way, it's likely the first photo you'll have of your little one. Attach a photo here to have as a focal point and a reminder of what your body is working toward.

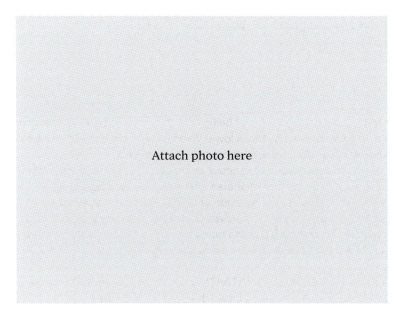

Attach photo here

#7

Exercise your options

Let's leap into the benefits of being ACTIVE, because there are tons to list. In general, exercise helps lower your risk of many chronic illnesses and improves sleep, energy, thought processes and anxiety. More specific to pregnancy, being active can reduce your risk of complications such as gestational diabetes, pregnancy-related high blood pressure, postpartum depression and common issues such as back pain. Keeping active also improves your odds of having a spontaneous vaginal birth, shorter labor and quicker postpartum recovery. In short: BETTER QUALITY OF LIFE!

Aim for 30 MINUTES OF ACTIVITY ON MOST DAYS, or 150 minutes a week. Most women can maintain their normal exercise routine throughout pregnancy, with some modifications as baby grows. However, MAKE SURE to discuss exercise with your medical provider first to be aware of any limitations specific to you. If you weren't exercising before becoming pregnant, try walking, swimming, exercise bands (for muscle strength), gentle yoga and/or beginner Pilates. Other tips:

- STRENUOUS ACTIVITIES can usually be continued if this was your norm prior to pregnancy. Remember to modify activities as your center of gravity changes with your pregnancy. Don't hold strenuous positions, hold your breath or have prolonged periods of lying on your back (particularly during the third trimester).
- TEMPERATURE CONTROL — Watch your environment and the humidity, and remember to drink water to hydrate.
- FYI: DIASTASIS RECTI (dye-AS-tuh-sis REK-tie) — Safe core strengthening may help prevent or limit this gap that can form in the center of your abdominal muscles. But, especially late in pregnancy, avoid heavy lifting and activities that put excess pressure on the abdomen, such as sitting up directly from a lying down position. (Roll to your side first.)
- KEGELS and SQUATS help strengthen your pelvic floor to gear up for birth and beyond! For Kegels, think of drawing up the pelvic floor muscles (not the glutes) toward your bellybutton like a core exercise, more than tightening them. Squats strengthen the leg muscles as well as the pelvic muscles.
- DAILY STRETCHING — Stability + mobility = a more comfortable mama. From the neck down to the feet, breathe deeply while doing gentle stretches to release tightness and stay spry.

#106

Field notes:
Pregnancy memories

Whether you're feeling the "glow" in pregnancy or you're sick of getting kicked in the ribs from the inside, leave some notes for future you and baby! You never know which memories of funny moments, little milestones or baby's quirks in the womb will fade with time. Use the prompts or write in your own.

Finding out and early pregnancy:

Notes on baby's activity (kicking, spinning):

Nausea and cravings and pains (oh, my!):

A fun or fascinating thing about pregnancy:

A less than fun thing about pregnancy:

Other memorable moments:

#8

The skinny on weight gain

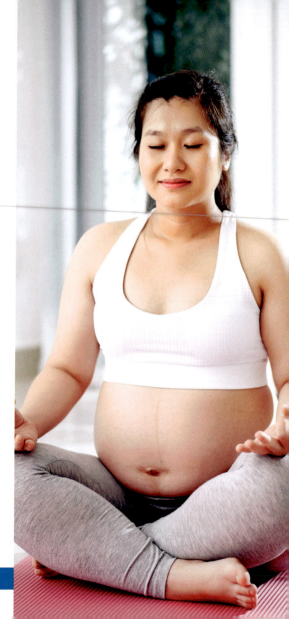

There are simple goals with pregnancy: healthy mom, healthy pregnancy, healthy baby. Weight gain is a part of that. Eat a variety of vegetables, fruits, whole grains, lean proteins and healthy fats — while limiting sugar, sodium and highly processed foods. If you do this, you'll likely gain within a healthy range. That makes pregnancy, labor, birth and recovery as easy as possible. It also makes it easier to lose the baby weight afterward.

REMEMBER THESE PRINCIPLES:

- Recommended weight gain is approximately 25 to 35 pounds if you are at a normal weight before pregnancy. If you're underweight or carrying multiples, the recommendation may be higher. If you have a higher body mass index (BMI), your provider may recommend gaining less.
- Almost half of all pregnant women gain more than what's recommended. Excess weight can make you uncomfortable, put you at risk of complications and possibly result in a bigger baby. These effects make pregnancy and birth more challenging, and they may increase the chance of a cesarean birth. Babies with a high birth weight are more likely to experience childhood obesity.
- Approximately 20% of women gain too little weight. This poses risks associated with baby being born smaller — tough start with feedings, easier to catch illness and possible developmental delays.
- In the first trimester, no additional calories are needed. In the second trimester, aim for an extra 340 calories daily, and an additional 450 calories in the third trimester. Think hummus and veggies and/or a healthy smoothie, not a triple-scoop ice cream cone. (Sorry!) TIP: Avoid bringing home junk food that will challenge your willpower each time you open the pantry.

#105

Feel enlivened

You crossed the finish line! Once you're home with your little one, trust in your knowledge to help you feel empowered and equipped. (And feel free to call your doctor or pediatrician for backup.) You've got this!

Scroll through this holistic list of universal ways to feel "enlivened." During the tough days or moments — as a new parent, as a partner, as a stressed-out human — these are key to keeping you healthy.

- EXERCISE — dance, walk, do whatever makes your body feel good.
- NOURISH — your body, mind and spirit.
- LAUGH — It causes physical changes that release endorphins, relieve stress, boost your immune system and actually improve your mood.
- IMAGINE — the good, the possible, the gratitude in your life.
- VOCALIZE — your feelings to a trusted friend, support group or therapist.
- EXHALE — deep, calm breaths.
- NATURE — Spend time near trees and/ or water. Going barefoot in the sand or grass may give extra benefits — it's called grounding or earthing and is rooted in evidence.

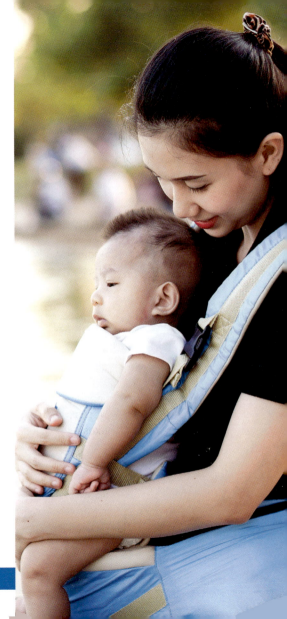

#9

Who will you see for prenatal care and delivery?

The where and the who of birth are very important decisions! See what providers and options are available in your community, and reflect upon your goals and medical needs. Which model fits your situation best? Do you need specialty care? Talk to people you trust.

IN-HOSPITAL BIRTH:
- Obstetricians — Physicians who are skilled at caring for both low- and high-risk pregnancies. When required, obstetricians (OBs) perform surgery. These doctors will also work closely with midwives and family medicine providers to help if needed.
- Certified nurse-midwives — Experts in low-risk pregnancies and births. Midwives are guardians of the natural process but can intervene when medically necessary to keep moms and babies safe. A midwife typically also makes every attempt to be present during labor when you need him/her most, as well as for the birth.
- Family physicians — Also experts in low-risk pregnancies. A bonus is their ability to care for the entire family, including baby after birth.
- Perinatologists or maternal-fetal medicine specialists — Physicians who specialize in caring for women who have complex medical histories or high-risk maternal complications. These doctors also care for pregnancies affected by fetal abnormalities.

OUT-OF-HOSPITAL BIRTH:
- Birth center — Typically staffed by midwives of varying certificates and licensure. Birth centers will have backup arrangements with OBs and hospitals in case a transfer needs to occur. Birth centers are an option for low-risk pregnancies.
- Home birth — Attended by midwives of varying certificates and licensure. This option should be considered only if your pregnancy is low risk. Be sure you understand the midwife's education level and experience, as well as the risks and benefits of home birth. You'll need a reliable plan in place in case an emergency hospital transfer is needed, which can still occur in a low-risk pregnancy.

Your choice of birth environment is just that — your personal choice. Some women feel more comfortable giving birth in an accredited birth center or hospital, while others prefer a planned home birth. Whichever you decide, know the benefits and risks of your decision.

Any of these options can give you a positive birth experience. A significant study found the greatest determining factors in a woman's satisfaction were the support and care she received during labor and delivery and being prepared for birth and possible complications.

#104

For the love!
(of your post-baby body)

- I STILL LOOK SIX MONTHS PREGNANT after having my baby — It takes six to eight weeks for your uterus to shrink back to its pre-pregnancy size. Breastfeeding triggers the uterus to contract. Eat healthy. Do some gentle, moderate exercise. Stay consistent and have patience!
- THERE'S A DARK LINE down my abdomen — It'll gradually fade over the next year, though it may not completely disappear.
- WILL THESE STRETCH MARKS FADE? — In time, yes (to an extent at least). Some people claim that creams and lotions during pregnancy and afterward help, although none has been shown to completely prevent or remove stretch marks.
- MY HAIR'S FALLING OUT — Your body hangs on to nutrients while pregnant and doesn't shed the 100 or so hairs each day that it normally does. You got to enjoy thicker, luxurious hair while pregnant, but for a few months after baby's born, you may notice extra shedding and/or thinning. It's normal. You could try hair-thickening shampoo or even cut your bangs to hide the sprouting hairs along your forehead hairline. (Check with your medical provider if you're still losing hair six months after delivery.)

- DIASTASIS RECTI — Typically this gap in the center of your ab muscles repairs itself over time, but you can help facilitate healing with gentle, core-strengthening exercises. A simple one can be done anywhere, in any position. During an exhale, think of "knitting" the lower ribcage together or lacing up an imaginary corset. The goal is to activate the abdominal muscles and narrow the torso while you exhale.
- INCONTINENCE — Kegels are pelvic floor exercises that help prevent or minimize the leaking of urine (such as when sneezing). Imagine stopping a stream of urine — the pelvic floor muscles are the muscles needed to do that. Aim for at least three sets of 10 reps/day, eventually holding some Kegels for up to 10 seconds. Squats also strengthen the pelvic floor (+ legs/glutes). Need more motivation for these exercises? Pelvic floor health and strength = better sex.

Try to be patient! Changes in your body may last many months as your organs shift back into place, your milk supply grows and stabilizes, and your tissues heal and strengthen.

#10

Doulas and labor support

One of the most important things you need for your baby's birth is SUPPORT! A doula is trained to provide physical, emotional and informational support to the mother and labor partner(s). Doulas don't perform any clinical or medical tasks. They typically meet with the parents a couple of times during pregnancy, offer continuous support through labor and delivery, and connect for a follow-up visit or two after baby's born. A doula will be your advocate and strive to make the experience of welcoming new life as close to your vision as possible.

CLINICAL STUDIES have found that women who have CONTINUOUS SUPPORT during labor are:

- Less likely to have a cesarean birth
- Less likely to use any pain medication
- Less likely to need labor induction, forceps or vacuum extraction
- Less likely to have postpartum depression
- Less likely to have babies who have a low 5-minute Apgar score (see page 50)
- More likely to result in shorter labors with fewer complications
- More likely to have success with breastfeeding
- More likely to rate their childbirth experience positively

MORE GREAT NEWS: All of these actually apply whether the continuous support is from a doula, companion or friend — it's just that most results indicate more benefit when a doula's present. If cost is a factor for having a doula, ask around! Volunteer doulas may be available in your local area. You could also ask if there are options for a reduced rate for a class or for auditing a training course.

If you want assistance after baby is born, postpartum doulas are specially trained for that. They can help guide you in how to take care of your baby and yourself as you recover, and can even lend a hand with some household tasks to ease the transition to parenthood. You can get connected with a doula by getting a referral from a care provider or trusted friend or by visiting a credible doula training program's website.

#103

Bonus points: Ways to save time and money

With all the added demands of parenthood, any saved minute or dollar can help!

WAYS TO SAVE TIME, ENERGY, $:
- Arrange a babysitting swap with good friends.
- For meals, make a double recipe and freeze half. (Or do meal swaps with a friend.)
- Order meal kits, and get ingredients delivered with recipes for simplified cooking.
- A grocery store near you may have options to preorder and pick up or deliver.
- Make smoothies for quick, healthy meals. (A good blender will even hide spinach! Try frozen spinach too.)
- Wear headbands or hats versus styling your hair.
- There's no shame in skipping a daily shampoo. (Those natural oils are actually good for shiny, healthy hair.) Try dry shampoo if your hair gets greasy quickly, and use a clarifying shampoo once a week if needed.
- Set up online bill pay through your bank account and skip all the check writing and mailing.

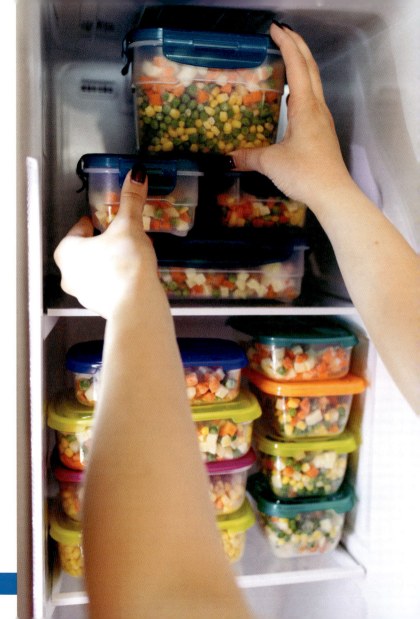

#11

Oh, the joys! Upper body common issues

Virtually every common discomfort of pregnancy is caused by hormonal changes and/or your body needing to compensate for a growing, space-occupying baby. Here's a brief list of some tried-and-true recommendations:

- MORNING/DAY/EVENING SICKNESS — Eat small, frequent meals so that your stomach doesn't get empty · stick to a bland diet · separate solids and liquids when eating · have someone else prepare your food · take prenatal vitamin later in the day and/or with food · use anti-nausea bands · rest · try acupuncture or acupressure · take vitamin B-6 · try ginger
- HEARTBURN — Eat small meals (slowly) · drink less during meals · avoid foods that are spicy, rich or fried · stay upright after eating · keep your torso lengthened · elevate your upper body when sleeping · avoid straining and heavy lifting · wear loosefitting clothing · take antacids as needed
- HEADACHES — Hydrate · rest · get a massage · take acetaminophen (Tylenol, others) · avoid migraine triggers if you're susceptible
- CONSTIPATION — Drink water · exercise · get fiber · eat veggies and fruits
- TINGLING/NUMBNESS IN HANDS — Limit repetitive motions · wear wrist splints at night
- BACK PAIN — Strengthen core muscles · wear an abdominal support belt to support the weight of a growing baby · apply heat · rest · massage · try physical therapy · seek chiropractic care

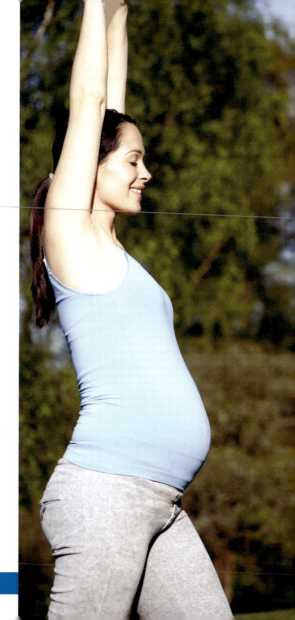

#102

Getting more sleep

Here are some gentle ways to promote sleep without tears (from your baby or from you):

- KEEP LIGHTS OFF or as dim as possible at night to prevent the brain from thinking it's time to wake up. Think room-darkening curtains to block moonlight and streetlights, turn your clock toward the wall, and so on.
- KEEP THINGS QUIET and limit talking during night wakings so baby doesn't think it's playtime. Also, silence phones whenever possible.
- SKIP DIAPER CHANGES overnight unless needed so babe stays sleepy.
- A BASSINET may be helpful to have next to your bedside so you don't need to get out of bed and become wide awake for night wakings or nursing. However, if you're breastfeeding, make sure to stay alert enough to return baby to the bassinet after nursing.

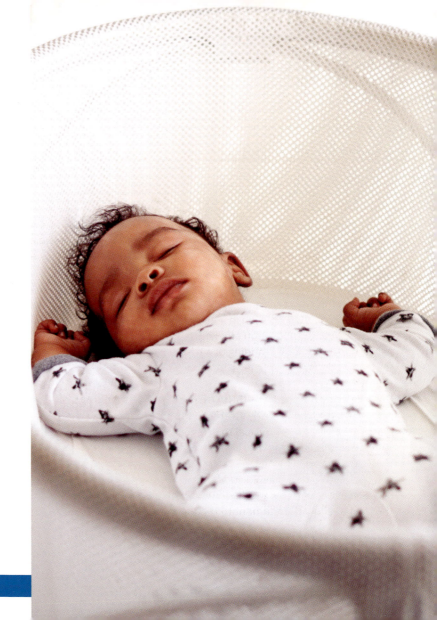

#12

Oh, the joys! Lower body common issues

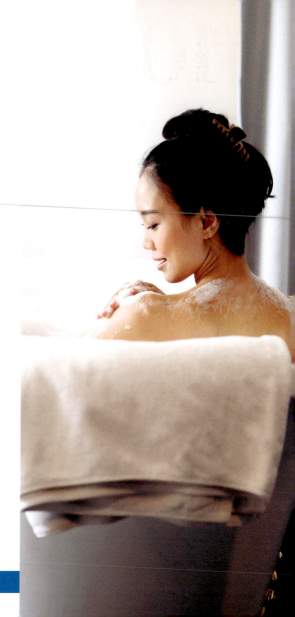

- HEMORRHOIDS — Prevent constipation · soak your bum in warm water · apply ice or refrigerated witch hazel pads to decrease swelling · avoid prolonged sitting and heavy lifting · try over-the-counter anti-inflammatory creams
- VARICOSE VEINS (common in legs and vulva) — Wear compression stockings · use cool packs · limit standing or sitting for long periods · elevate legs · exercise regularly
- PAIN IN LOW BACK/BUTT (SCIATICA) — Apply heat and ice · gently stretch leg and gluteal muscles · try physical therapy · seek chiropractic care
- ROUND LIGAMENT PAIN — Gently stretch sides and abdomen · avoid sudden movements · lean toward the direction of the pain to allow the ligament to relax

- LEG CRAMPS — Stay hydrated · gently stretch calf muscles before bed · take warm baths · try extra magnesium and calcium
- SWOLLEN FEET/ANKLES — Wear compression stockings · keep legs elevated when you can · stay hydrated · avoid salty foods · soak in the tub · go swimming · walk
- RESTLESS LEGS SYNDROME — Take iron supplements if advised for low iron level · exercise, do yoga, stretch and walk · massage the legs · wear compression stockings during the day · decrease caffeine · take warm baths before bed

#101

Bring on the bliss

Baby's fed, burped, changed, rested. Check. Here are a few more tricks that can help minimize fussing:

- CUES — Respond to nonverbal cues from baby to keep the happy vibes going longer. (Review page 54!) Babies whose needs are met sooner tend to cry less.
- BABYWEARING — Consider keeping your baby close in a carrier, sling or wrap. Having your hands free isn't the only benefit! The familiarity of being warm and snug, all that motion, and hearing a heartbeat and voices can help baby feel secure. To stay safe, follow guidelines for infant weight and possible time limits for your specific carrier. Additional safety checks: Baby's mouth and nose stay uncovered for breathing. Baby doesn't get too warm. Baby is positioned where you can easily see his or her face. Baby's knees should be higher than the bum so that spine and hips are supported for healthy development.
- SWADDLING — Your newborn may love being wrapped like a burrito — which can promote calmness and sleep. Arms can be swaddled (until there's a risk of baby rolling over) or free to suck on hands to self-soothe. Safety checks: Make sure baby is back sleeping. Don't let your newborn sleep through needed feedings. Watch for overheating. Also, make sure there's room for those little legs to move easily for proper hip development.
- PLAYTIME — Right away, your brilliant baby may start imitating certain facial expressions. Make an O with your mouth or stick out your tongue — the entertainment begins. The best "showtime" is when baby is quiet and alert, not drowsy or active.
- CULPRITS — If your little one seems inconsolable after feedings, talk with baby's medical provider. Tricky conditions such as reflux, heartburn or colic might be causing discomfort, or the underlying cause might be a food sensitivity (such as to dairy or soy) or an overactive letdown of milk that overwhelms baby.
- SKIN-TO-SKIN CONTACT — Keep skin time going through the early weeks for bonding with both parents.

#13

Dental care

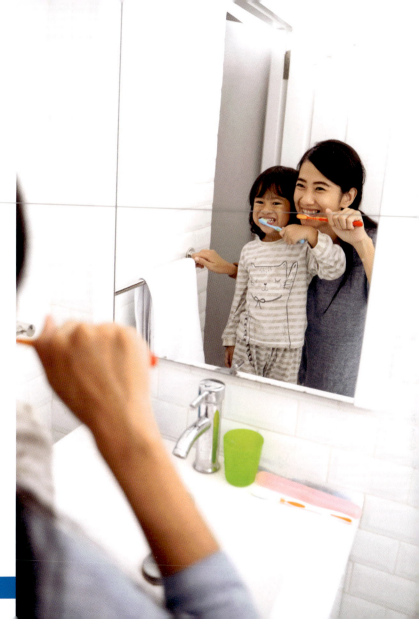

FLOSS ONLY THE TEETH YOU WANT TO KEEP!

Growing a baby may be tiring, but don't neglect your personal hygiene. During pregnancy, increased acidity in the mouth raises the risk of tooth decay. In addition, the surge of hormones in pregnancy can make gum tissue more prone to gum disease. Plaque contains millions of bacteria, and this sticky film needs to be brushed off. Plaque along the gumline can harden into tartar and increase the risk of gingivitis. If gingivitis is left untreated, it can lead to periodontitis — and a mouth that's really aching, to say the least. Prevent, prevent, prevent. BRUSH AT LEAST TWICE EACH DAY and after meals or sugary treats and drinks when possible. FLOSS and USE MOUTHWASH DAILY. And get dental CHECKUPS EVERY SIX MONTHS. Don't be alarmed if you have a little extra bleeding when flossing. This is a result of increased blood volume during pregnancy.

And always inform your dentist that you're pregnant, so your treatment plan can be modified if needed.

#100

Reminders for labor support

Generate an attitude of confidence, compassion and peace:

- ENCOURAGE.
- Be in tune.
- READ HER NEED.
- Use cool washcloths, warm words.
- RESPOND ASAP TO HER REQUESTS.
- "Hold space" for mom.
- SUPPORT (physically as well as emotionally).
- Be a consistent source of calm reassurance — through each contraction, each change of position, each push.

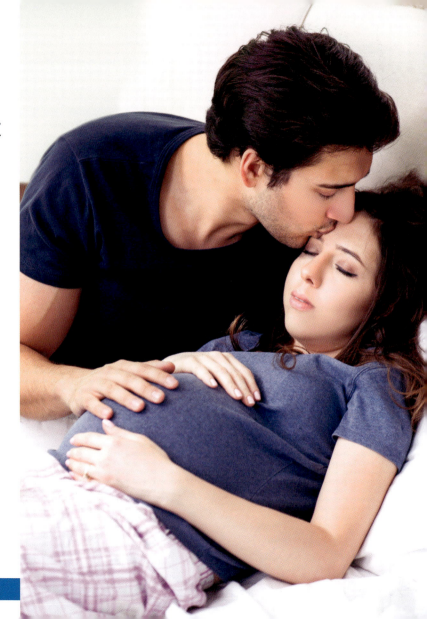

#14

Home sweet homeostasis

HOMEOSTASIS IS BEING IN A RELATIVELY STABLE STATE OF BALANCE WITH YOUR MIND AND BODY. HOMEOSTASIS IN MOM HELPS CREATE AN OPTIMAL ENVIRONMENT FOR BABY TO GROW IN.
Help you and your baby thrive by AVOIDING EXTREMES in these areas as best as possible:

- STRESS — A high level of stress isn't good for you or your pea in the pod. Learn what calms you down, and do it whenever life escalates. Educate yourself about the practice of mindfulness and seek out local classes, podcasts, books or online videos. Breathe deeply, be in nature, exercise, listen to music, chat with a good friend, serve others, watch a comedy or relax with a cup of tea.

- TEMPERATURE — Babies can't regulate their temperature on the inside. Your baby is relying on you for climate control, so it's best to avoid or limit hot tubs, saunas and strenuous exercise in very hot or humid weather while pregnant.
- FLUIDS — Drinking water during pregnancy is crucial for several reasons. Staying well hydrated decreases swelling (edema) and your risk for bladder and kidney infections. It helps prevent uterine contractions from dehydration. Need more convincing? It also helps bowel function and helps prevent constipation, which can lead to bloating and hemorrhoids. (And, conveniently, staying hydrated helps regulate internal body temperature, which makes it easier for your body to endure stress.)

- CIRCULATION — There has been a long-held belief that lying on your left side was the best during pregnancy, and back sleeping was a no-no. Research now shows that there is no difference in adverse pregnancy outcomes regardless of your sleep position — at least through 30 weeks. After that time, it's likely still best to avoid lying on your back for long periods. The baby's weight is increasing and could cause compression of a large blood vessel that runs along your spine. Listen to your body! Women haven't always had a book telling which positions to avoid. If something doesn't feel right (like lying on your back with a large baby in your belly), don't do it. If you wake up on your back, simply readjust.

#99

Phrases mama might appreciate hearing

- You're doing it!
- You ... are ... strong.
- You'll be holding your baby soon!
- Everything is going just as it should.
- You amaze me.
- I'm so proud of you!
- You're making awesome progress.
- Thank you for all the work you're doing!
- You are so much stronger than this contraction. (Or substitute wave, rush or surge. See page 92.)
- Release that wave. (Use after a contraction.)
- Soothing words such as *peace, relax, comfort, calm, impressive, admirable, gratitude, hope, joy.*
- Follow me ... (for example, when mama is breathing too fast and could use some guidance on breathing more slowly and calmly).

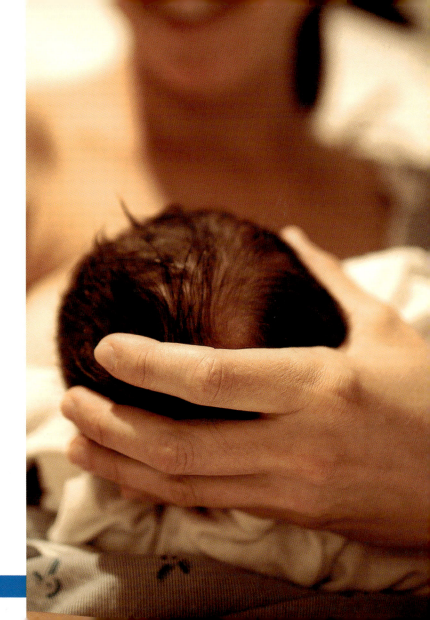

#15
Mentally strong

Truth: A predictor of good mental health after baby is born is to have it BEFORE baby is born. It's completely understandable why your emotions may be heightened during your pregnancy and postpartum. Know that you're not alone and that it's not your fault. During your pregnancy, do what you need to do to feel empowered! Here are some ways to cultivate feelings of being mentally strong:

- Limit your use of the internet and social media. If you have a question about your pregnancy or health, ask your medical provider or use reputable resources.
- Practice yoga, mindfulness, meditation and/or prayer.
- TALK to your partner, family and friends. Make sure those who are closest to you understand that you may be struggling a bit.
- Eat a healthy diet! Get adequate rest and daily exercise (even just walking). Spend time outdoors.
- SHARE changes in your mood with your provider. He or she is there to help you.
- Consider cognitive behavioral therapy. This helps give you awareness of your negative thoughts and teaches you to respond to them in a productive way.
- Remember that medication is an option. Any potential risks can be discussed with your medical provider, but many medications for anxiety and depression are safe during pregnancy and breastfeeding.

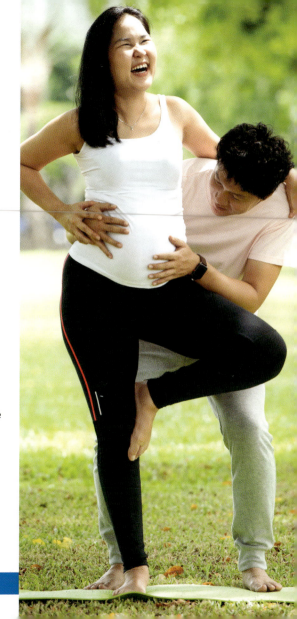

#98

Words of strength

Focusing on a single word or a short series of
words can help you get through a contraction.
Here are a few we recommend you try:

BREATHE

RELEASE

LOVE

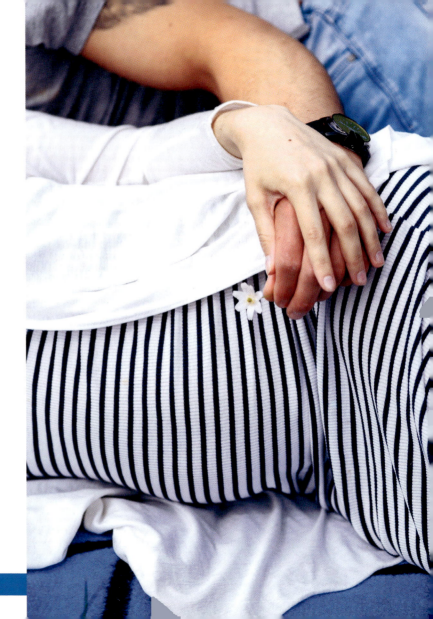

#16

Writing your birth plan/ preferences

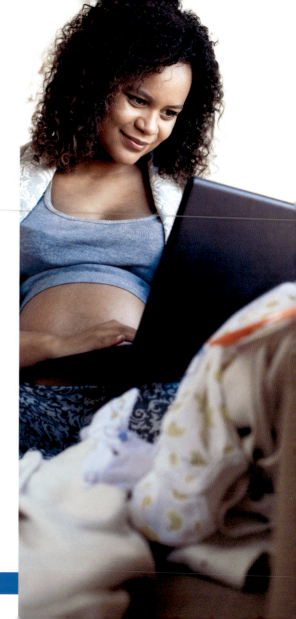

Let's face it: Birth is unpredictable and can't be totally planned for. Get your labor team on the same page with a guide to how you'd like to be cared for throughout your birth and postpartum time. Things to keep in mind:

- KEEP IT BRIEF — Your hospital or birth center may give you a form to fill out. If not, make your birth plan one page. Using bullet points is A-OK. Include a short introduction of yourself, a section on what you'd like for the birth (Pain relief? A mirror to see delivery? Who should be present?), and desires or questions about postpartum and newborn procedures (Are skin-to-skin and delayed cord clamping routine? Which vaccines are given and when?).
- KEEP IT REALISTIC and RELEVANT — Do all you can before you go into labor to prepare for the birth you'd like, learn what your hospital or birth center will allow, and learn what procedures may be suggested.
- KEEP IT POSITIVE — Try to limit the use of "no" or "unless absolutely necessary," as the medical situation will determine which procedures are needed to keep you and baby safe. If you're worried your care provider may perform an unnecessary procedure, you may want to consider switching to someone more aligned with your goals. Keep in mind that if you're working with a team of providers that rotates who's on call, some may not be as acquainted with your preferences.
- REVIEW the plan with your care provider and labor support team ahead of time.
- BE YOUR OWN ADVOCATE — If your provider recommends something such as starting medications or placing internal monitors, ask questions until you understand why. Discuss the risks, benefits and options, and if the situation could be closely monitored and given time to resolve.

#97

Conqueror

"After two false alarms to labor and delivery triage, I was finally admitted after a 1 centimeter change in my cervix. I was filled with a thousand emotions: excited, nervous, worried, happy and sad. Fear suddenly took over. Within an hour, an epidural was placed and my pain and anxiety started to diminish. My labor progressed unpleasantly slowly. The doctor had to break my water, expecting good progress after that, but my contractions were still weak. I only dilated about ½ to 1 cm every hour, and some hours none. Talk about a defeating mental game! Pitocin was used in my IV to help speed up my labor. On top of this, my daughter had her first bowel movement in the womb, so meconium was seen in the amniotic fluid. Her heart rate decreased frequently, especially if I was on my back, so I needed to stay on my sides. Since I had an epidural, I needed to be moved by the nurse.

"A long 24 hours later, I was finally ready to push! I ended up pushing on my hands and knees to help with the decelerations of my daughter's heart rate. This was difficult because of the epidural — but it worked. Two hours later I was able to feel my daughter's head of hair, which gave me extra motivation. Soon, the NICU team arrived. My daughter was delivered and placed on my chest. The NICU team then evaluated her, and they suctioned her lungs deeply because of the meconium.

"I delivered an almost 10-pound baby vaginally, with a very minimal tear! Although my labor was difficult, I wouldn't change it for the world. Not only do we have a healthy baby girl but I was also able to conquer the mental and physical challenges of labor — which has only made me stronger."

#17

Don't leave home without …

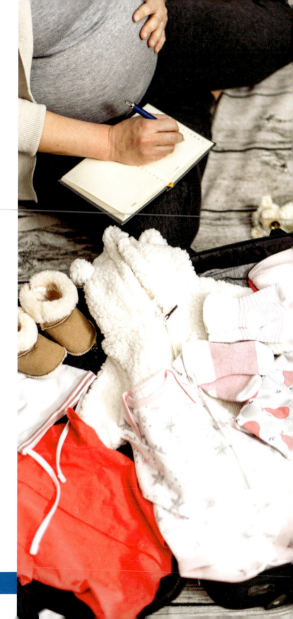

Birth works best when you're comfortable and relaxed, so include these items in your hospital bag:

- YOUR OWN CLOTHES — Stretchy nightgowns or skirts for labor · a layer with short sleeves to easily check blood pressure · socks · robe · slippers · swimsuit · comfy, loose pants (to accommodate large pads) for postpartum · underwear · necklines convenient for nursing · nursing bra
- RELAXATION TOOLS — Music · aromatherapy (if allowed) · battery-powered candles · massage oil or lotion (unscented might be preferred in labor)
- MOTIVATIONAL TOOLS — Special photo · a focal point to keep your eye on the prize
- SNACKS — Best to refuel in small increments: soft fruit · applesauce · oatmeal · broth · granola bars · trail mix

- TOILETRIES — Toothbrush and toothpaste · glasses/contact supplies · deodorant · hair bands · makeup · lip balm · breath fresheners
- TECHNOLOGY — Camera · video camera · cellphones · tripod · chargers · extra camera batteries
- PAPERWORK — Any hospital forms · photo ID · insurance card · copies of your birth plan
- KEEPSAKES — Extra paper or card stock for footprints
- FOR PARTNERS — Supportive shoes · comfortable clothes with layers · money for parking and vending machines · a foldable, hand-held fan for some hero moments during labor
- FOR BABY — Car seat · going-home outfit · baby blanket
- And this book for motivation and reminders during labor

#96

What truly matters

"My husband and I didn't have our birth plan written in stone, but one thing was certain: We wanted to avoid a cesarean. When a cesarean became reality as the best option for a SAFE and HEALTHY DELIVERY of our baby and for MY WELL-BEING, we recognized we had no choice.

"The decision in the moment was the easy part. The harder part happened in the weeks that followed when I had to grieve the fact that I was not able to have a vaginal birth. I struggled with thoughts of, what's wrong with my body? What's wrong with me? Why could I not do this natural process? What would have happened if medicine was not advanced enough to allow for a cesarean as an option?

"I had to ALLOW MYSELF TO GRIEVE, and then had to forgive myself and LET GO OF THE THOUGHTS of how things should be and instead focus on what was. We were blessed with a BEAUTIFUL, PERFECT, HEALTHY BABY girl — and that was what truly mattered."

BIRTH STORIES

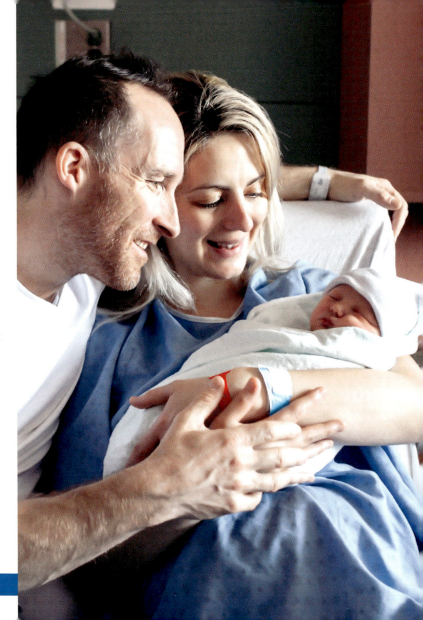

#18

Get ready for birth

Although impatience to meet your babe can be overflowing at the end of your pregnancy, remember that baby and hormones are what trigger labor to begin. Unless medically indicated, allow for those last stages of development and growth, and don't rush the process. Until late in the game, baby's lungs are still maturing, the immune system is strengthening, and iron is being stored to meet baby's needs for the next six months or so. Baby is also adding fat and developing mechanisms needed to maintain body temp.

Here are some ideas for activities to help pass the time:

- MOVEMENT — Walking, swimming and prenatal yoga can be especially helpful. The Cat-Cow, for example, is a gentle stretch to prevent/relieve low back pain, strengthen abdominal muscles and improve circulation. Some birthing gurus encourage being on your hands and knees several times a day, in particular during the last four to six weeks of pregnancy. This may be doing exercises or even reading a magazine on all fours. But limit prolonged sitting and reclined positions (lie on your side instead). Many experts insist that these movements can facilitate getting baby into an optimal position, which typically leads to a faster and less painful labor. BINGO!
- TALK — Voice your fears and anxieties about labor, birth and becoming a parent. Birth is a mental game as much as anything else, so mamas sometimes need to get in the right mindset before labor will unfold.
- REST and NOURISH YOUR BODY in preparation for birth and motherhood. Tie up loose ends at work, eat healthfully (and put some extra meals in your freezer for after baby comes), and get plenty of sleep.
- BODYWORK — Chiropractic, acupuncture, and/or massage can help you stay comfortable.
- SEX — Many women wonder what can help start their labor. Is there anything? Unlikely. Think of this as a protective factor. You wouldn't want a normal, daily activity such as walking or eating a common food, such as pineapple, for instance, to start labor too early. Having said that, one activity shows some potential: SEX. Although most evidence says it won't help, some studies have shown that it may reduce your need for induction of labor at 41+ weeks.

#95

Gratitude

"I went in for my 39-week checkup, and the doc was concerned our baby's growth had plateaued. I was to be induced at 8:00 the following morning. Long story short, it took a draining day and a half for the Pitocin to really kick in.

"Here's a list of some unexpected detours we took: being induced and having an epidural, a resident delivering our baby, an episiotomy (the resident's first), a team waiting to make sure our baby was safe (they faded into the background) and our little bundle being taken to the nursery due to low blood sugar when he was only a few hours young.

"Our adorable baby boy weighed 5 pounds, 11 ounces. We interlocked gazes and focused only on him and our immense gratitude. It was the middle of the night, so we didn't interrupt this sacred time with even one phone call till morning.

"Our little guy also needed to stay a few days longer in the hospital, which was scary. BUT ... this allowed me time to learn how to take care of a newborn. By the time we brought him home, I felt much more competent as a mom. I was actually euphoric — for months. In retrospect, I think the key factor was having so much support from the caring resident, my incredible husband, family and friends ... and one particular nurse who took me under her wing."

#19

The squeeze

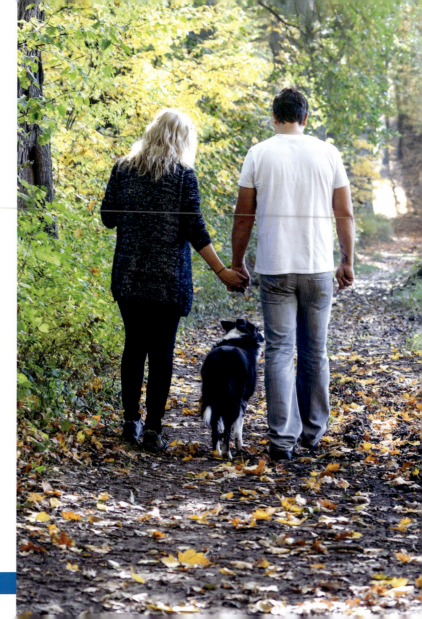

Knowing if birth is right around the corner can be confusing. Even seasoned mothers may be unsure since each pregnancy experience can differ from a previous one.

- YOUR UTERUS may contract A LOT at the end of a pregnancy, with some discomfort. If you're feeling contractions and it's 10 p.m., take a warm bath, snuggle in and go to bed. Staying up until 3 a.m. counting contractions that ultimately cease = one tired mama. We promise you will not sleep through labor.
- WHAT DO YOU WATCH FOR? Think of the word *progressive,* meaning contractions that consistently get closer and more regular over time — and, most importantly, get stronger, stronger, stronger.
- MOMS FEEL CONTRACTIONS DIFFERENTLY. They may be high, low, in the front, in the back, wrapping around the body or in one steady spot.
- DON'T BECOME OBSESSED with counting and monitoring. The regularity and strength of the squeeze will grab your attention.

#94

Hello, gravity

"Our final change of position was the winner. My husband sat on the side of the bed and I squatted between his legs, resting my arms and elbows on his legs as he supported me. HELLO, GRAVITY! My pushing became so productive and rewarding in this position. I could feel baby moving down through my body and the building pressure on my bottom. After a few pushes, I put my hand down and could feel baby's head right there!"

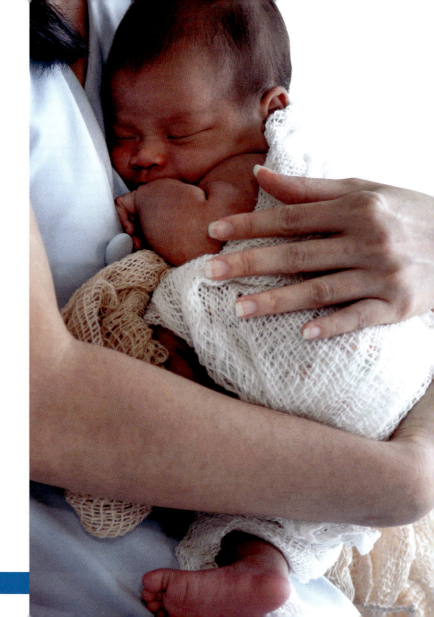

#20

Other than contractions, what else should grab your attention?

COMMON SIGNS that labor may be getting close include general discomfort, feeling low/menstrual-like cramps, thigh pain, back pain, loose stools, increased nesting and feeling under the weather. Also watch for:

- WATER BREAKING — Persistent, tiny trickling of water ... or more like Niagara Falls splashing down to your feet. (Either way, water breaking may not happen until later in active labor.) Regardless of quantity, call your medical provider and report on "COAT":
  - C — Color of the fluid
  - O — Odor
  - A — Amount (trickle or gush)
  - T — Time of rupture or release

- MECONIUM-STAINED AMNIOTIC FLUID — This explains the C for "color." Sometimes babies poop before they're born, which makes the leaking amniotic fluid greenish in color. This is more common when pregnancies go past 41 weeks. If you notice this issue, your care team will watch baby's heart rate more continuously in labor, and experts from the neonatal intensive care unit (NICU) will likely be ready to intervene in the rare situation that your baby has respiratory problems.

- DECREASE IN FETAL MOVEMENT — Although baby's movement may be more subtle (vs. jabs and kicks) at the end of pregnancy, you should still feel regular fetal movement. ALWAYS let your provider know if you're concerned that your baby isn't moving as much as usual.

- LOSING YOUR MUCOUS PLUG — A big glob of mucous certainly will grab your attention! It may be yellow or blood-tinged from blood vessels that break as the cervix changes in preparation for birth. It's a good sign that things are changing, but no indicator as to when your baby will be born — it could be hours or even a couple of weeks.

- BLEEDING — When you're in labor, having bloody show — discharge of blood-tinged mucus when blood vessels break as the cervix opens — is normal. Talk to your medical provider right away if the bleeding seems abnormal or concerning.

#93

Rerouting to reach the same destination

Maybe you've envisioned your birth story with excitement and anticipation. Often, the mental pictures of labor that you hold may display flawless behavior and control — a labor that starts and progresses exactly how textbooks describe and a beautiful vaginal birth after 20 minutes of pushing. Pooping and perineal tears? No way.

But what happens when things don't go as planned?

- As with all aspects of life, few births go exactly as envisioned or desired. Expect some detours. If you can start with this attitude, you're less likely to be disappointed in your birth experience if it's not "perfectly executed." No matter what happens — it's still YOUR UNIQUE birth story.

- Arm yourself ahead of time with education. Attend birth prep classes, and read and reread the practical tips in these pages. For some real talk, ask trusted friends and relatives to share their favorite memories and helpful advice from their birth stories.

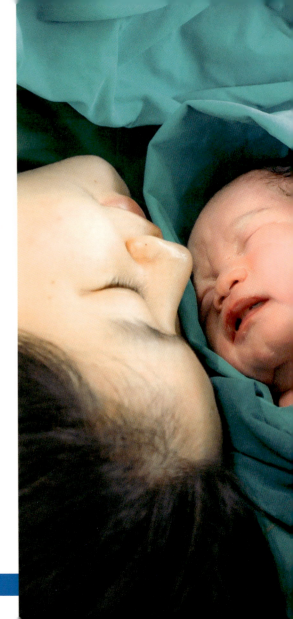

#21

GO time!

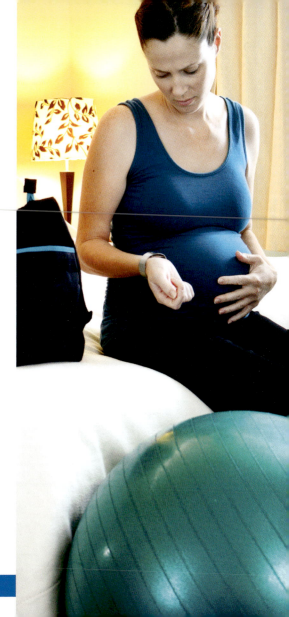

WHEN TO HEAD TO THE HOSPITAL OR BIRTH CENTER

Deciding when to head to the hospital can be tricky, but look for any of these signs to know when it's time:

- CONTRACTIONS GETTING LONGER, stronger and closer together — The exact timing isn't as important as the change in the intensity and consistency of the pattern. If you or your birth partner is timing the contractions, note that how far apart they are is measured from the start of one contraction to the start of the next.
- THE 'LABOR ZONE' — When a laboring woman loses her ability to be a conversationalist and is instead very focused (often with added moans and/or deeper breathing).
- THE 'FEELING' — The laboring woman's desire to be in the place where her baby will be born.
- THOUGHTS ABOUT THE CAR RIDE — The speed of labor can't be predicted for anyone, even if it's your first baby. A ride to the hospital isn't always an easy one (driver included!). Do your very best to plan this trip BEFORE it seems to be an overwhelming one. Don't forget to take weather and traffic into consideration, and keep enough gas in the car so you won't have to make a pit stop.
- SPECIAL SITUATIONS — Most advice in this book is for a healthy, full-term pregnancy (37 weeks and beyond). Your own situation or care provider may prefer you to labor very little at home.

#92

Ride the 'wave'

The words you use in describing an experi-ence — contract, constrict, tighten, pain — can cause an undesired response in your body. Give yourself some options using different terminology and see if it creates a helpful shift in perspective. For example, you could refer to a contraction as a RUSH, WAVE, SURGE, PRESSURE, SENSATION or INTENSITY. This shift in mindset can lead to a positive shift in your body and improve the entire experience of birth.

You can also try rephrasing these terms:
· Labor = birthing time
· False labor = practice waves or rushes
· Dilation = opening
· Transition = transformation, about to meet baby
· Delivery = birthing

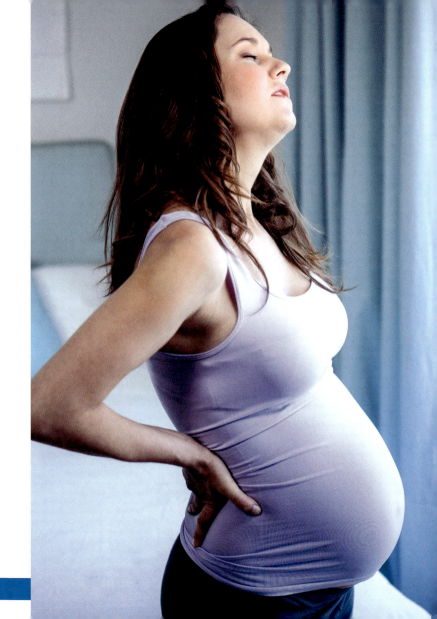

#22

Keep these in mind throughout labor

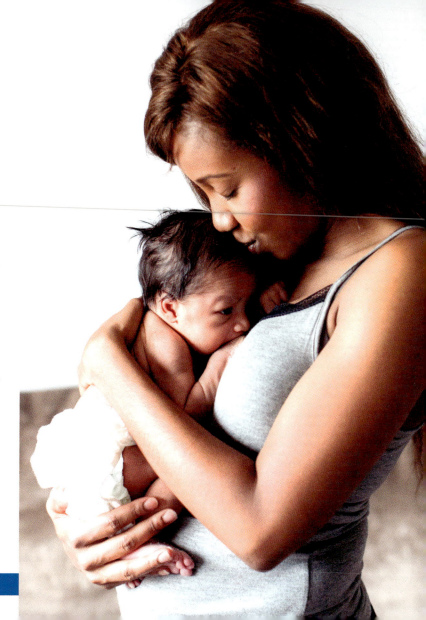

- TRY TO CHANGE COMFORT MEASURES every hour or so — more often if needed.
- URINATE EVERY HOUR or two to keep the bladder empty, which will give baby plenty of room to move down plus help the uterus work more efficiently.
- THINGS ARE ALWAYS CHANGING. What works now may not later, and what didn't work before, may now.
- ALTERNATE between restful and active comfort measures as needed.
- Birth partners: Ask for FEEDBACK BETWEEN CONTRACTIONS, and offer suggestions such as, "Really let your jaw relax even more." During contractions, try to allow mom to stay in her zone.
- VISUALIZATION, encouraging words and a positive attitude are fantastic tools!
- BE PROUD of each and every step you make.

DURING LABOR

#91

Set labor goals in baby steps

During labor, take things one contraction at a time, just as a runner might focus on only one mile at a time.

SET SMALL, INCREMENTAL GOALS, such as "I'm going to do three more contractions in this position and then try something different" or "I can do this for 15 more minutes and then reevaluate."

Often, things shift. By the next increment, baby moves, your perspective changes and energy can be renewed and refocused to keep running the race.

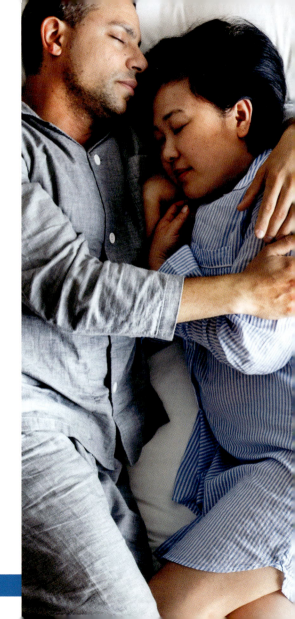

#23

The pain paradigm

THESE CONCEPTS ARE USEFUL THROUGHOUT LIFE, TOO!
You may have heard the phrase "Pain with a purpose." In labor, this purpose goes beyond the incredible goal of holding your baby. There's far more occurring during labor and delivery than what the eye can see. For example, pain can nudge you to move in ways that help labor progress. Pain helps the body produce oxytocin and endorphins, which help regulate contractions. And pushing baby down the birth canal helps squeeze liquid from baby's lungs. Keep all this in mind, and know that pain is a normal part of the birth process. If it helps, you can reframe it by referring to it as pressure.

One important distinction is pain versus suffering. They are not the same. Your support team should take great care to help keep you from suffering.

Here are THREE EFFECTIVE WAYS TO COPE with purposeful, productive pain:
1. Central nervous system control — You can reframe your perception of pain and how it's interpreted by the brain. The goal is to stay in the calm, parasympathetic nervous system rather than activating the sympathetic nervous system and its fight-or-flight response. Childbirth education, continuous doula support, relaxation and music all can help you to reframe the perception of pain.

2. Gate-control theory — The gist of this complex concept is that flooding the nerves with nonpainful sensations reduces the painful signals that get through the "gate" to the brain. Nonpainful sensations can even scoot through the gate first. Think of hurting your finger and then holding it, rubbing it or shaking it. Examples in pregnancy and labor include gentle massage, movement, warm packs and water immersion.

3. Diffuse noxious inhibitory control — This can be described as "pain inhibits pain." Think acupressure, deep massage, deep counter pressure and sterile water injections. The painful stimuli trigger the release of endorphins, which are morphine-like hormones. Pretty nifty.

Using a combination of these three methods, customized to mama's preference, may be the most effective approach.

#90

Trust

TRUST YOUR BODY. It's beyond brilliant!

TRUST YOUR BABY. More often than not, he or she knows what to do.

You've chosen your MEDICAL PROVIDER wisely, so be confident in his or her skills.

Make sure your BIRTH PARTNER knows that if you feel well supported, you'll be better able to allow your body to take over rather than wanting to be in control. This may make it easier to cope throughout your pregnancy, too.

SURRENDER TO THE PROCESS, and know that the end result will be worth all you've endured!

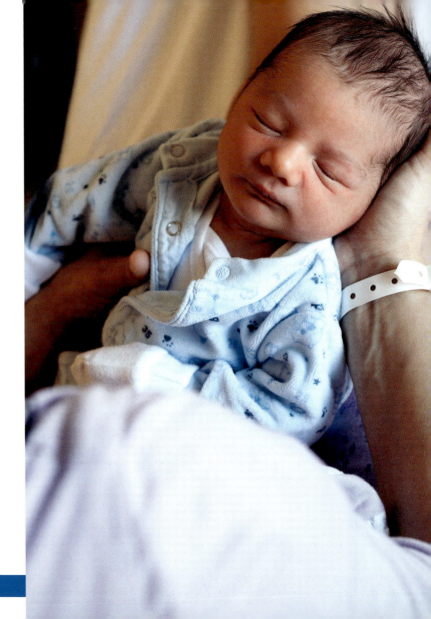

#24

Stay relaxed

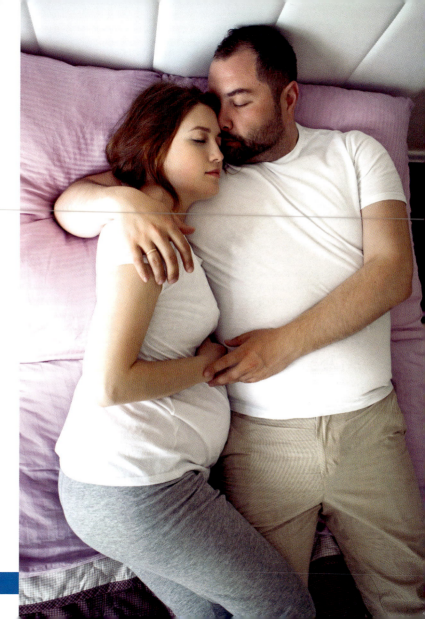

Relaxation is the key to coping with labor. When you're stressed or anxious, you become tense — just the opposite of what's needed during labor. This tension leads to pain, which perpetuates the cycle. This ultimately can cause a slowing of labor. Practice relaxation techniques leading up to labor, so you'll be able to conserve energy, prevent and alleviate pain, allow for better oxygen supply to baby, and keep labor progressing. Try these tricks:

- Have a slow, even BREATHING PATTERN.
- Do a mental scan of your body — brow, jaw, shoulders, fists, buttocks, thighs, feet — to RELEASE TIGHTNESS. Let that tension flow right out of your body.
- THINK OF WORDS such as *soften, release, melt, open, loose, peaceful, floating, safe, supported, heavy, down* and *ease*. Focus on what resonates with you — it may be waves, a flower opening, the circles that ripple from a water droplet or something else you dream up. Practice at night when you're falling asleep, and your body will be more trained to do this in labor.

#89

Near the end of your pregnancy

Almost every mom begins to feel impatient at the end of pregnancy. The excitement to see what baby looks like, feels like and smells like has been building for a long time. In addition, fatigue and normal discomforts contribute to wanting to be done with pregnancy. Not to mention the question you may get asked repeatedly: "When is that baby coming?"

Tips to help you cope:
- Follow through on some nesting urges to make your physical environment more comfortable for when you come home with baby. It will keep you moving — and can have a positive ripple effect emotionally.
- Think of your due date as more of a due MONTH. Mentally, this is much better than watching the calendar and counting on baby to be punctual. More than 50% of pregnancies go past their due dates.

- Remember: Waiting for labor to start may take patience. Inducing labor is sometimes necessary and safest. But if you find yourself wishing for an induction or your medical provider offers it, talk about the pros and cons. Some research has suggested that there may be benefits to inducing women at 39 weeks versus waiting for natural labor. But expert opinion varies, as research findings can't be generalized for all women or be reproduced on all labor and delivery units.
- Treasure these final moments with your current family. Get cozy on the couch, have lingering conversations, and enjoy the peace and quiet of your home. LIFE IS ABOUT TO CHANGE.

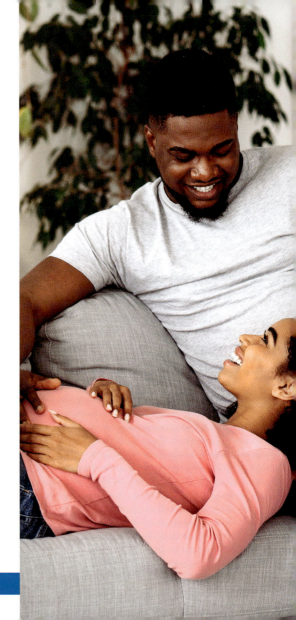

#25

Labor positions

To get baby into a good position for birth, it helps to keep mom moving. So walk, sway, rock and change positions frequently. Staying upright — except when you need to rest — may allow gravity to assist you and your babe. Note: You can be seated or kneeling and still be upright.

- STANDING — Moving around while standing causes changes in pelvic joints, which can facilitate baby moving down the birth canal. Try walking, slow dancing, lunging or leaning forward.
- ALL FOURS — Try resting your upper body on a birth ball, bed or tub.
- SQUATTING — It vastly widens the pelvic outlet, shortens the birth canal and provides a mechanical advantage with the upper trunk pressing downward. (You may want to lean forward or stand between contractions.) Keep your heels down on the floor, if possible, as being on tiptoe tenses muscles. Try alone, supported or using a squat bar in a birthing bed.
- SITTING — Use a rocking chair, birth ball, bed, toilet or birth stool, or semirecline. Feel free to adjust the hospital bed to find your position of comfort.
- LUNGE — Elevate your front leg on a bed or stable chair, toes and knee of the elevated foot turned out. Slowly lunge forward in the direction of your foot and hold the stretch for a few breaths, then return upright. Alternate legs every few contractions. A kneeling version can be done lunging to the side. Just keep the lunging foot on the floor rather than elevated.
- KNEELING — Rest your upper body on a bed, chair or birth ball.
- LYING DOWN — Position yourself on your side with pillows between your knees to open your pelvis. Place a pillow under your belly and one behind the back for support. Alternate sides periodically.

Whether you're seated on a birth ball, on all fours or standing, find your inner hula — try moving your hips and doing figure eights to keep things moving.

#88

Be gentle, forgiving and patient with yourself

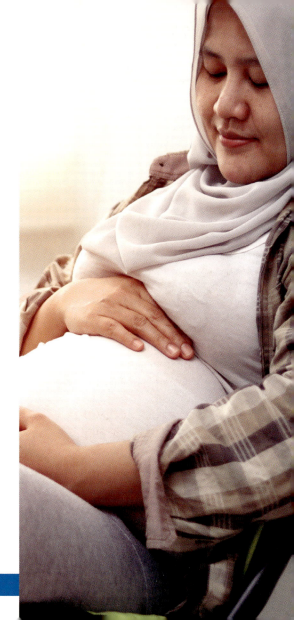

WHILE YOU'RE PREGNANT

- Your BLOOD VOLUME INCREASES 40% to 50%, and all the abdominal organs are shifted to make room for the growing baby. (No wonder a flight of stairs leaves you winded when it didn't before!)
- Your circulatory system sets up hundreds of new capillaries to accommodate the increased blood flow in your body.
- Your ligaments — especially in the hips, abdomen and pelvis — become overstretched to accommodate your growing baby. This causes the joints to become loose or unstable. That, along with hormone changes, is the reason for the PREGNANCY WADDLE.
- Recommended weight gain is typically 25 to 35 pounds but could be higher or lower for you. This is bound to change how your body feels and looks.
- THE UTERUS IS THE MOST TRANSFORMATIONAL MUSCLE IN THE BODY, as well as one of the most powerful muscles. And it's getting the workout of a lifetime.
- Throughout pregnancy and early postpartum, your body RAMPS UP ON ESTROGEN, PROGESTERONE AND OTHER HORMONES. The result? So many possible effects, including heightened emotions, feeling short of breath, constipation, increased vaginal secretions, skin changes, and an increase of varicose veins in the legs and vulva.
- Above all, remember that this is what your body is designed to do. Pregnancy and birth are normal.

Normal, but not always easy. Be as gracious with yourself as you'd be with a close friend!

#26

Set the mood

Here's a thought: Birth is a little like sex. It involves the same female body parts and hormones, so it stands to reason that the desired environment for birth might be a personal, intimate setting. You may want the room to include:

- DIM LIGHTING
- Your preference of MUSIC
- AROMATHERAPY, if allowed at your birth place
- Battery-powered CANDLES (open flames = fire danger)
- QUIET, calm voices
- FEW INTERRUPTIONS
- Your own comfortable, SOFT CLOTHES and fabrics

Or instead of a private setting with only your partner, you may want the loving support of generations surrounding you! You choose.

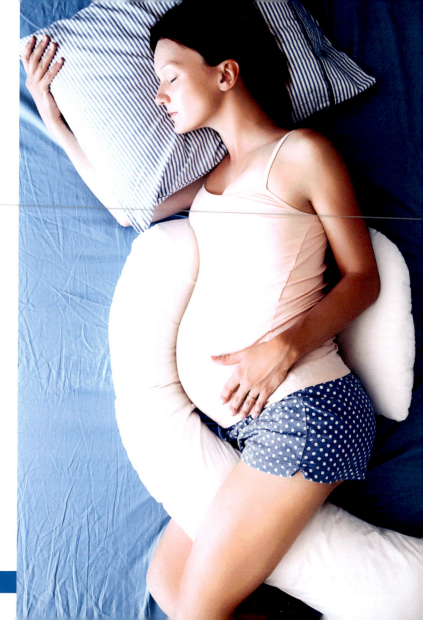

DURING LABOR

#87

Rebuilding your immune defense after antibiotics

If mom needs to take antibiotics during pregnancy or labor, baby is also exposed to the antibiotics. Antibiotics wipe out good bacteria as well as the bad. It's extremely important to rebuild the good bacteria, because they help defend the body against harmful pathogens — especially in the gastrointestinal (GI) tract. A healthy GI tract in children is needed for the absorption of nutrients, which enables them to grow optimally and can impact long-term health.

WOW #1 — An estimated 70% of your immune system is actually located in your gut!

WOW #2 — Most of your body's serotonin (hormone involved in mood control, depression and aggression) is produced in your digestive tract.

WAYS TO IMPROVE GUT FLORA:
- Limit sugar. (See how much your body thrives when you keep sugar to 25 grams or less per day.)
- Limit processed, refined foods and drinks.
- Eat fermented foods like sauerkraut, kefir and fermented vegetables (pasteurized versions are the safest).
- Watch the ingredients — many yogurts are loaded with sugar, artificial sweeteners and coloring, and actually have LOW levels of beneficial bacteria.
- Take a quality probiotic.
- Breastfeeding is extremely beneficial for baby's immune system.

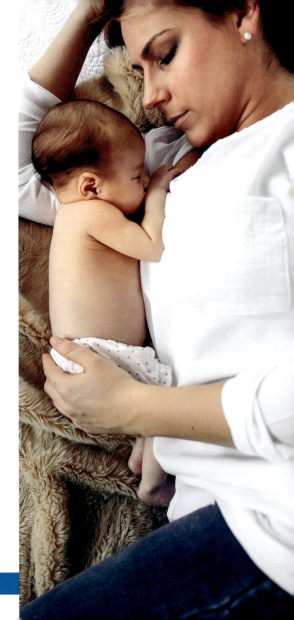

POTENTIAL DETOURS FROM YOUR PLAN

#27

Cool it, baby!

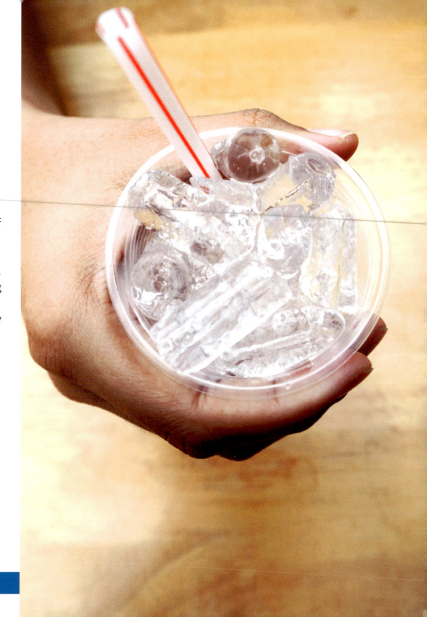

Cold provides a distraction from contractions, in addition to pain relief through the temporary numbing and cooling qualities it provides to a hot, uncomfortable mama. Try these things to cool off:

- Apply COLD WASHCLOTHS to the forehead, neck, chest and back. Plan to get a bowl full of ice water and several washcloths, changing out for a fresh cold one with the beginning of each contraction.
- Toss a couple of cans of soda in that same ice bath and use to apply COOL PRESSURE to a sore lower back. Roll the cans to massage.
- Keep ICE WATER handy, preferably in a cup or bottle with a straw to offer easy hydration between contractions.
- ICE CHIPS = deliciousness in labor. It may sound cliché and a little crazy, but noshing on ice chips has been a longtime favorite of laboring women around the world.

#86

Cesarean (C-section) birth

There are important reasons why a family might need or desire a cesarean birth. However different your ideal birth might look, a cesarean is still the amazing birth of a baby ... YOUR amazing birth of YOUR baby.

- SHARE YOUR BIRTH PREFERENCES with your surgical team to determine what you CAN still have for your birth (for example, delayed cord clamping, skin-to-skin contact, a doula).
- The operating room (OR) will be bright and may be chilly, with machines and sterile supplies. The team will help you get positioned on the OR table.
- There may be several medical providers in the room, some unfamiliar, all with masked faces: nurses, anesthesia staff, the pediatric team and OB providers.
- The anesthesia team will be most visible to you, at your head. They are THERE TO KEEP YOU SAFE and ensure that you're comfortable.
- A drape will be placed on your abdomen that will also rise high above your head, about 6 inches in front of your face.
- You may feel fear, excitement, nausea, apprehension, relief, cold and/or shaky.

- Your labor support (usually just one) will be brought to you once the team is assured that you can be awake during the cesarean (meaning the spinal/epidural is working). That person will be seated right near your head. DON'T FORGET THE CAMERA!
- You should feel no sharp pain — only pressure and tugging. In a very short time, voila! Your baby will emerge! The OB team may give you a sneak peek as the drape is briefly lowered, and then hand baby to the pediatric team to quickly assess. Your support person can stay with baby and take pictures, ogle, touch.
- Assuming that you and baby are both doing well, have baby placed on your chest, even while your incision is being repaired. If you're not feeling up to it, your support person can hold baby near you. Babies are usually wide-eyed and quiet at this time, so PEACEFULLY REST, CHEEK-TO-CHEEK, SKIN-TO-SKIN, and get to know your baby. With the proper help, breastfeeding could even be initiated.
- After surgery is complete, you'll move to a recovery room for about two hours, where you can continue skin-to-skin and breastfeeding. Congratulations on your birth!

POTENTIAL DETOURS FROM YOUR PLAN

#28

Warm it up

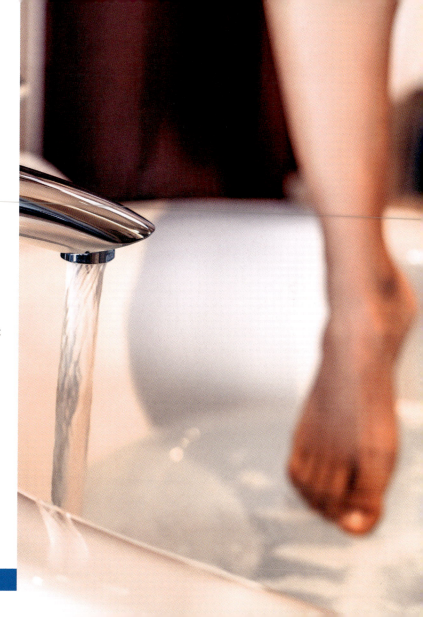

Use of heat in labor stimulates a favorable biomechanical reaction within the body that promotes relaxation and calmness and soothes sore muscles. Ways to bring on the heat:

- Place A WARM PACK on the lower back, neck or belly. Ask if your place of birth has warm packs or if you should bring your own. Filling up a tube sock with rice or flaxseed makes a fabulous warm pack. Use a microwave to heat it up gradually. Be careful that it's not hot enough to burn your skin, which is why some hospitals don't offer them.
- SOAK IN A TUB or stand or sit in the shower with warm water flowing on your body.
- Ask for WARM BLANKETS at the hospital or heat your own at home in the dryer.

#85

Some potential interventions

It's completely normal to feel nervous or disappointed when labor doesn't go as planned. Remember that multiple factors are assessed and considered when doctors and midwives recommend interventions.

- INDUCTION OF LABOR — Sometimes labor needs to be initiated. Reasons include being late term (41 to 42 weeks) or a specific medical complication where it's determined that baby is better off out than in. Methods of induction vary and depend largely on mom's cervical exam.
- INTRAVENOUS (IV) FLUIDS — During an uncomplicated labor, routine IV fluids are not typically necessary, and it can limit mobility. But if you are having a hard time keeping up with fluids by mouth, IV fluids may be recommended. (Ask if intermittent use would be possible too!)
- AUGMENTATION OF LABOR — This involves the need to speed up the process

a bit, even if mom is having regular contractions. It can be accomplished by breaking the bag of waters, use of IV Pitocin or nipple stimulation.

- INTRAUTERINE RESUSCITATION — Sounds scarier than it really is. If baby has persistent heart rate decelerations or other concerns, there are things that can be done to mom that will positively affect baby, including:
  - Position change — Turning mom from side to side or on her hands and knees can take pressure off an umbilical cord that's temporarily getting squeezed.
  - Oxygen — It provides an extra boost to the placenta, helping baby get a bit more too.
  - IV fluids — They also provide an extra boost to the placenta, especially if mom has become dehydrated.
- AMNIOINFUSION — This intervention replaces fluid around the baby by using

an IUPC (intrauterine pressure catheter). The added fluid can help to cushion the umbilical cord if it's getting pinched (common during contractions) and baby's heart rate is repeatedly having decelerations.

- OPERATIVE VAGINAL BIRTH — This is achieved by use of vacuum or forceps, depending on the situation and preference of your medical provider. It may be recommended if the provider needs to assist or expedite vaginal birth due to maternal exhaustion or fetal heart rate concerns.
- CESAREAN BIRTH — Situations that typically call for (indicate) a cesarean include stalled labor progress, baby not descending with pushing, fetal heart rate concerns, breech position, planned repeat cesarean birth or rare occurrences that put mom or baby at risk.

#29

Get wet

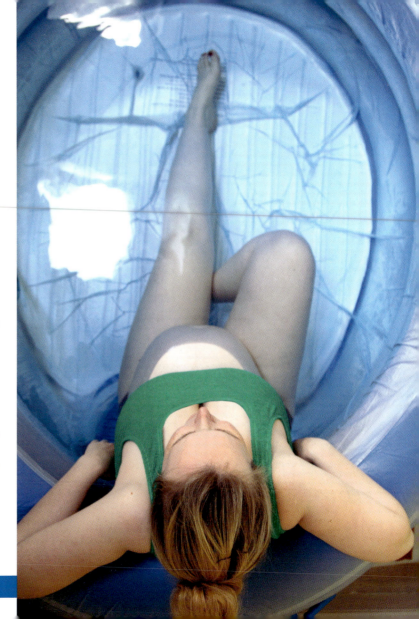

Your baby is hanging out in water, so maybe you should, too! Water can be an amazing tool for all stages of labor. Give one or all of these a try:

- BATHS — A warm bath can help you relax in labor. But, even better, laboring in the tub has other proven benefits! It can be helpful for pain relief and, hence, has been shown to decrease the use of pain medications. It may even help to shorten your labor. Being tucked in the water with no apparent risks to baby can also provide an added sense of privacy. While in the water, continue to move and change positions and stay well hydrated. Hop out as needed to cool down, rest or keep moving.
- SHOWERS — Many hospitals have a detachable shower head. Use it to help you massage your back, belly and shoulders.
- WARM OR COLD COMPRESSES and WASHCLOTHS — Have them handy for whenever. They can be especially soothing near the end of labor and while pushing to help the perineum stretch (warm water for that). Ask your medical provider or labor nurse to help out.

#84

Wrong way, baby!

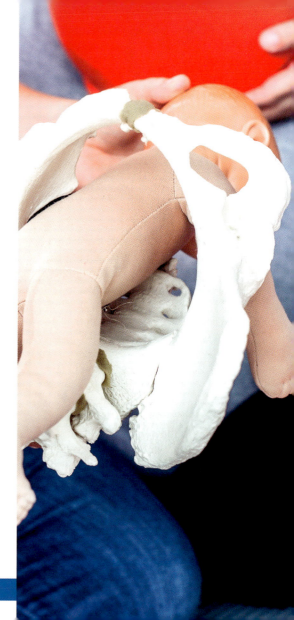

- BREECH — Approximately 3% to 4% of babies are either butt or feet first at the end of pregnancy. Even less common, babies can be lying crosswise (transverse). These positions occur most commonly in a mom who's had several babies, has polyhydramnios (lots of amniotic fluid = extra room to swim) or whose uterus is abnormally shaped. Around 36 to 37 weeks, medical providers will assess whether the baby is head down.
- OCCIPUT POSTERIOR ("OP" or "sunny side up") — Ideally, when a baby descends into the pelvis, the head/chin should tuck and baby should be looking down toward mom's back. When a baby is OP, he/she is facing front. The typical result: a longer labor, "back labor" felt in the low back and increased risk of needing forceps/vacuum/cesarean birth. Mom should change positions frequently in labor. Side-lying, elevating one foot on a stable chair and lunging toward it, or hanging her belly down while on her hands and knees are possible ideas. If an OP position persists and is affecting baby's descent with pushing, your medical provider may be able to rotate baby's head manually.
- ASYNCLITIC — Baby's head may be tucked, but it is tilted a bit to one side or the other, making for a difficult fit. The typical result: a longer labor and increased risk of a cesarean birth. Again, mom should change positions frequently, trying to facilitate baby to self-correct. Fencing-like lunges to the side with the front leg on a chair may be the answer. Do this on both sides, alternating every few contractions.

#30

Energize

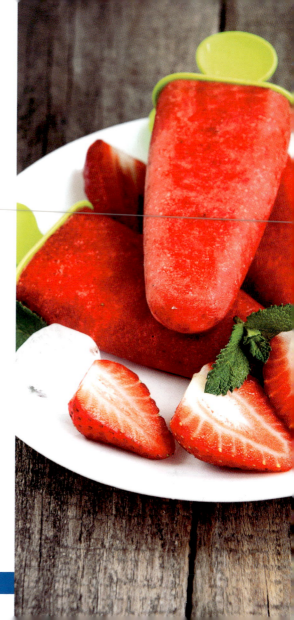

They don't call it labor for nothing — having a baby is hard work. Incorporate these energizing techniques into your birth plan to help keep up your strength and reduce fatigue:

- EAT — While you may not want a full meal, eat light snacks and take quick bites to stabilize your energy level. Frozen juice pops offer quick energy as well as cooling. Ask if your hospital or birth center would be able to keep them in a freezer for you.
- DRINK WATER — Drinking between contractions = staying hydrated = a well-functioning uterus and placenta = smoother labor for mom and babe. Another bonus: The movements of going to the bathroom — squatting and releasing the pelvic floor — can help the baby wiggle into birth position. Try urinating at least every couple of hours. If you're able to, it's a good sign you're staying hydrated.
- GET SOME AIR — No matter the weather, fresh air can bring a fresh perspective and energy to your labor.
- TAKE A SHOWER — It's a great way to wake up and recharge. Even just splashing cool water or spritzing water on your face can help perk you up.
- TRY AROMATHERAPY — Scents like orange, lemon and peppermint can give you an energy boost. Ask what forms of aromatherapy are allowed at your birth center. Due to allergy concerns, some hospitals have restrictions.

#83

Making it through the birth canal

The birth route is ... incredible. If that's not the word you would use, these facts may give you a whole new appreciation for the birth process.

- As baby passes through the birth canal, baby's lungs are squeezed to help REMOVE FLUID remaining in the lungs that was necessary during development, but now needs to be removed to breathe.
- Why do some babies have a bit of a cone-shaped head right after being born? Slow travel through the birth canal can be helpful for mom and baby as baby's skull shifts to make the journey south.
- In the womb, the baby's gut is sterile. As the baby passes through the birth canal, IMPORTANT "GOOD" BACTERIA are picked up from mom that help develop baby's underdeveloped immune system as it faces the challenges of a new environment. The bacteria also aid in digesting breast milk, reducing colic and improving gut health, potentially for years.
- To add to that thought, studies have shown that children born vaginally have a lower incidence of obesity, asthma and autoimmune diseases — all of which are associated with changes in the microbiome. It's also a fact that the microbiome is very different between babies born via cesarean versus born vaginally. Researchers are still exploring how the birth pathway may affect long-term health, so stay tuned. Meanwhile, remember that a cesarean birth is sometimes the best option to give mom and baby a healthy start on this new adventure!

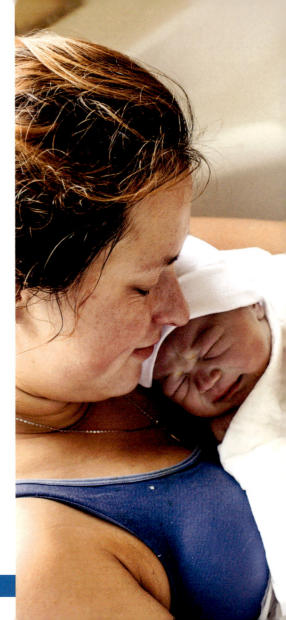

#31

The 'zone'

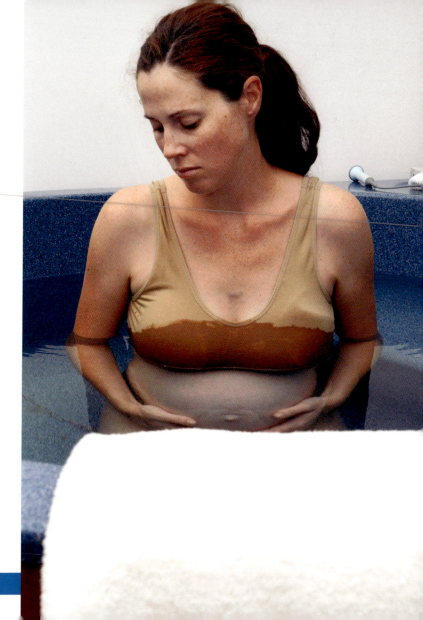

There are points during the labor process when you may find that coping with labor becomes more difficult, and self-doubt creeps in. This might occur:

- When moving from early labor to active labor (see page 61) as contractions become closer and stronger.
- If active labor has taken a toll, and you feel weary.
- During transition, late in active labor as the body prepares for the pushing and birth phase. Transition can be intense, but it's typically the fastest part of labor. You're on the home stretch (literally)!

The secret to coping during labor is to FIND YOUR ZONE. The zone is different for everyone, but the meaning is the same. It's finding your inner strength by utilizing some type of practice that provides distraction or laser focus. The practice may be a visualization, a verbalization, something auditory or a combination of all of these. See the following pages for examples.

#82

Holy hormones

There are many hormones at play throughout the journey of pregnancy, birth and breastfeeding. The following four key players are the most influential. No need to dig out your notebooks from science class, just appreciate the power of hormones — and, more importantly, recognize how your thoughts can direct your emotions and hormones. Biology's got this.

- OXYTOCIN — The "hormone of love," oxytocin is released whenever hanging out with loved ones, giving or receiving a hug, and during orgasm, for example, to give an overall feeling of well-being. It also causes contractions of the uterus during labor and contractions of the milk-producing cells during lactation, leading to the milk ejection reflex, often called let-down.
- ENDORPHINS — Similar to morphine and heroin, endorphins provide pain relief plus an altered state of mind in labor. This allows moms to cope with contractions while tapping into their primal, birthing instincts. Feel-good endorphins are released alongside oxytocin, contributing to balance and coping abilities in the labor process.
- CATECHOLAMINES — These include dopamine, epinephrine (adrenaline) and norepinephrine (noradrenaline). They're released during stressful situations, times of anxiety and anytime the basic needs of survival — food, water, safety — aren't being met. They inhibit oxytocin release, which means if you have catecholamines in your birth, they could reduce the effectiveness of your contractions and affect progress in labor.
- PROLACTIN — If you've got prolactin, you've got milk! And the good news is, levels of this milk-making hormone start to build by the end of the first trimester and continue to rise throughout pregnancy to ensure you'll have plenty of milk for your baby when he or she arrives. This hormone also helps you put baby's needs first, hence the nickname "the mothering hormone."

#32

The zone via strength of mind

Made-up statistic: Birth is 90% in your head and 10% in your body. Really, though, the mind has the power to overtake the work of the body and impact labor in a positive or negative way. Keep yourself in the right mindset by using these tricks:

- Have an INSPIRATIONAL VERSE, mantra, prayer, chant, song or person you admire to think about.
- Take a MENTAL TRIP to a favorite place, happy time or peaceful memory. Your body will follow.
- Think about a SIGNIFICANT ACCOMPLISHMENT or time when you felt empowered.
- ENVISION HOLDING and snuggling your kiddo!
- Know that whatever roller coaster of emotions you ride during labor is rewarded by the greatest feeling of RELEASE.

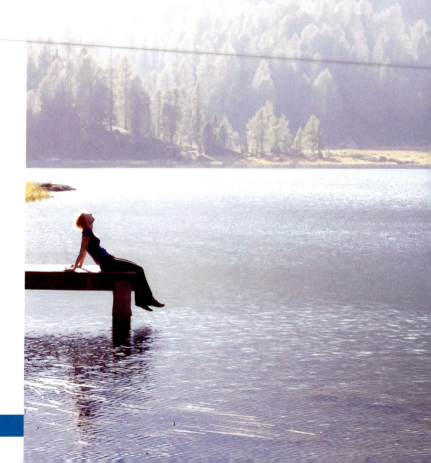

#81

FYI: Speaking of epidurals

Let's review the benefits and risks of an epidural for pain relief.

BENEFITS:
- Epidurals can provide effective pain relief and help an exhausted mama get good rest.
- If a cesarean birth is required, an epidural may be used to give additional medication so that you can be awake during surgery.
- Epidurals are helpful in the rare event of a stuck placenta or the need to repair extensive tearing of the perineum.

RISKS:
The overall risks of having an epidural are very low. They may include:
- A longer pushing phase and an increased need to assist birth with forceps or vacuum tool, which is more likely to cause perineal tears.
- It's common for your blood pressure to decrease, potentially causing you to feel lightheaded and nauseated, needing meds or additional IV fluids for control. This could compromise oxygen supply to baby, and this leads to the next point.
- Sometimes a baby's heart rate can decrease shortly after an epidural is placed. This could be related to a drop in your blood pressure or is sometimes due to sudden hormonal changes after quick pain relief. This shouldn't lead to a need for a cesarean birth or long-term concerns with baby.
- Spinal headaches, which occur after only about 1% of epidurals.
- The epidural may be uneven and be less effective on one side. About 9% to 10% don't work perfectly.
- Fever can occur, especially if the epidural has been in place for several hours. The kicker here is that it's difficult to tell the difference between an epidural fever or one from an infection in the uterus. Given this, maternal fever in labor often forces the diagnosis of a uterine infection and the start of antibiotics. This could also mean blood draws and antibiotics for baby. A fever increases the chance of cesarean birth.
- Itchy skin is a very common, minor side effect.

Note: An epidural usually limits the free movement that's helpful for labor progression. If you're planning on getting an epidural, focus on what you can do BEFORE you have it placed. Walk, lunge, be upright on the ball, get in the tub, and MOVE as much as you can. This is especially true for first-time moms, whose labors are often longer.

#33

The zone via a focal point

Concentrate on a specific object during every contraction.
A-n-y-t-h-i-n-g that catches your eye and keeps you focused.
Examples include:

- FAMILY PHOTO or wedding picture or pictures of kids, cats or dogs
- The FACE of your partner or labor support person
- BABY CLOTHES or blanket for going home from the hospital, to help the surreal feel real
- CARDS with positive birth affirmations — make your own or ask a craft-loving friend to help
- A MIRROR to see progress during pushing or to watch your baby being born
- A SPOT ON THE WALL — if it catches your eye, feel free to use it
- A WORD or series of words to serve as your mantra

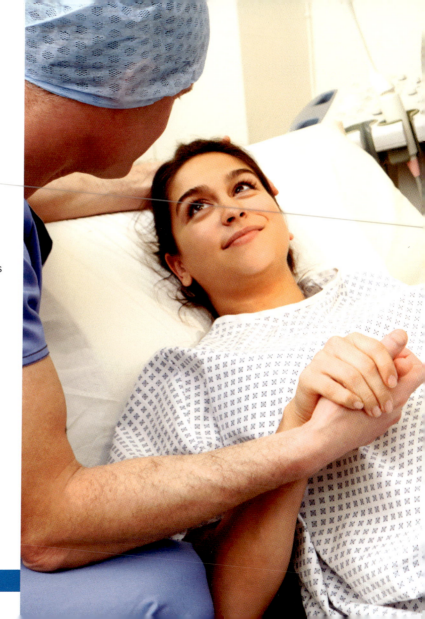

#80

Pain relief medications

Maybe you're planning to take advantage of modern pain relief options during labor, or maybe you'd prefer to go without. Either way, it's smart to be aware of your options, in case circumstances change. Getting baby safely into your arms is what really matters!

Things to know:
- INDUCED LABOR, prolonged labor or required interventions may contribute to changing plans for natural childbirth.
- Typical options include opioid pain medications, nitrous oxide or an epidural:
  - OPIOID (aka narcotic) — It takes the edge off the contraction, making the peak feel less strong. It will also help you relax more between contractions. A very small amount of these medications will pass to baby, possibly causing a drowsy effect. Because of this, providers try not to give opioids if birth is soon approaching.
- NITROUS OXIDE — Inhaled through a patient-controlled mask, it can help reduce the intensity of pain almost immediately. (Ideally, start inhaling 30 to 45 seconds before a contraction.) Adverse effects are typically minor. Check with your provider to see if it's an option.
- EPIDURALS and spinal anesthesia — These options provide the strongest pain relief. They are more invasive, with medication injected into or near the spinal canal to block pain in a large region. They typically require additional interventions such as an IV, bladder catheter and continuous fetal monitoring. (See page 81.)
- DISCUSS YOUR MEDICATION OPTIONS including choice, timing, risks, benefits and alternatives of pain medications with your care team (labor nurse/doctor/midwife/birth partner). Your given situation may dictate which option is best for you.

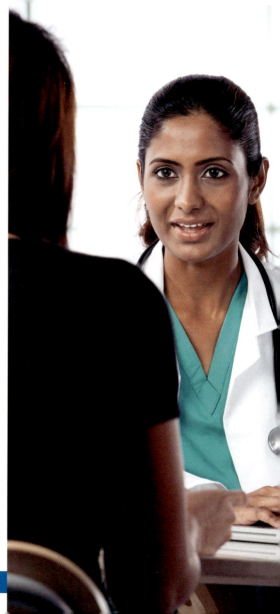

#34

The zone via the power of sound

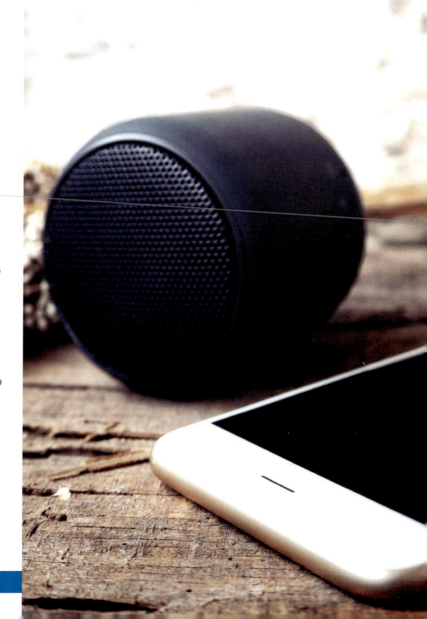

Sometimes birth is loud. Sometimes it's quiet. The important thing is to find what works best for you to feel calm, while also having the freedom to release tension. Some good noises include:

- LONG, DEEP MOANS — from your gut — during the exhale breaths when there's a contraction. Focus on the sound of the moan and the vibration you feel at the back of your throat. It's relaxing for you and your baby. Have someone do it with you if you're feeling self-conscious.
- BIG SIGHS, noisy "horse-lip" exhales, or even roars. Don't be embarrassed by the primitive sounds or chants that may escape your mouth. Birth is an instinctual part of the human experience, so it's only normal to make some noise.
- COUNTING. One … two … three.
- MANTRAS. You might try "Ooooopen," "Ouuut" or "I can do it!" Experiment with different words or phrases.
- The VOICE OF YOUR SUPPORT PERSON or team.
- A good dose of LAUGHTER can do wonders! Reminisce about funny stories with those around you. It provides a nice distraction and will make those endorphins — the body's natural "feel good" hormones — surge.
- Your FAVORITE MUSIC. Whatever rocks your world!

#79

Monitoring mom and babe during labor and birth

The job of your midwife or doctor and labor nurse is to be guardians of your care. It means keeping a watchful eye and intervening when medically necessary. These tools of the trade are common for monitoring labor:

- Fetal monitor with Doppler ultrasound (intermittent or continuous) — Although not perfect, it's currently the best tool to assess the pattern of the fetal heart rate, which gives providers a cue as to baby's well-being. Frequency of monitoring depends on maternal risk factors, how the baby is tolerating labor, and/or if baby has passed stool (meconium), making the amniotic fluid greenish in color. An internal monitor may be placed if baby needs to be watched closely and external monitoring isn't optimal. IMPORTANT FACT: Over the years, continuous fetal monitoring has increased the cesarean section, forceps and vacuum rates. It's helped improve the rate of neonatal seizures, but has NOT decreased the risk of cerebral palsy.
- "Toco" for contractions — The external toco, short for tocodynamometer, measures only the timing and length of contractions. If your provider needs to know the actual strength (because of prolonged labor/cervix not opening), then a special monitor may be placed during an exam. This flexible tube lies alongside baby and measures the actual pressure of the contractions.
- Cervical exams — Checking the cervix for dilation or change is typically done to see if labor is progressing normally. These exams should be done as a standard of care — not out of pure curiosity. Exams can increase the risk of infection and can be uncomfortable. Generally speaking, the cervix is checked every four hours in earlier labor and every two hours during active labor. Of course this varies based on each mom's situation — whether it's less or more frequent.
- Vital signs — They're monitored to assure that mom's blood pressure, heart rate and temperature stay within the normal range.
- Other labs — They're most commonly done if mom has gestational diabetes or blood pressure concerns.

Note: If continuous fetal monitoring is needed, ask if a portable telemetry unit is available so mom can be more mobile during labor.

#35

Coping with back pain:
Part 1

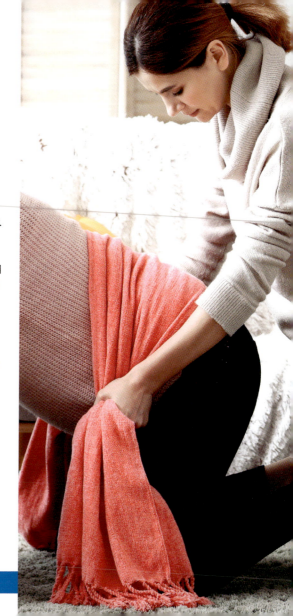

Back labor — feeling all the pain of the contractions in the back and none in the front — occurs in 25% to 30% of labors. It typically, but not always, happens when baby isn't in the optimal position, or when mom has a pelvic anomaly or previous injury. Labor often progresses slowly with back labor, as the baby has to work harder to find the easiest path out. Comfort measures include:

- DOUBLE HIP SQUEEZE/PELVIC PRESS — See page 40.
- COUNTERPRESSURE on low back — Use your hands, fists or a massage tool (see page 41).
- HEAT/COLD — Use a hot-cold pack or small bucket with ice water and stack of washcloths for your back, neck or face.

- HYDROTHERAPY — Take a bath or shower. Use a removable showerhead to massage the back.
- ROLLING PRESSURE — Try rolling a chilled soda can, a frozen juice can or a tennis ball in a sock (easier to hold and maneuver) on your low back.
- STERILE WATER INJECTIONS — Shallow injections of sterile water are placed just under the skin of your low back. These feel like a big, bad bee sting going in, but can help relieve low back pain for up to two hours, and they involve no medications. Ask your medical provider if this is an option for you.

#78

Additional prenatal tests and screenings

The following tests might also be recommended. While they may provide further information about your baby's health, they aren't necessarily 100% accurate. Your medical provider can discuss with you the purpose, benefits and risks of these tests.

GENETIC CARRIER TESTING (typically done before or early in pregnancy):
- Carrier screening can detect genes associated with a wide variety of genetic disorders (for example, cystic fibrosis) that could be passed on to your child. Screening for some of the most common variants is routinely offered, even if you don't have known risk factors. Risk factors include family history or specific heritage that's more commonly associated with certain genetic disorders.

GENETIC PRENATAL SCREENING:
- Screening tests are available in pregnancy that can help screen for the likelihood of a chromosomal issue in baby. Mom's age and the personal and/or family history of both parents can be risk factors. These tests may consist of just bloodwork for mom or an added ultrasound. Some have to be done in a specific time frame during pregnancy. Genetic screening has pros and cons, and whether to have it is a personal choice. In addition to talking with your medical provider, you may find it helpful to meet with a genetics professional.
- If any screening test is positive, further investigation — typically an invasive prenatal test — may be able to provide a more certain diagnosis. Your provider will discuss the options and risks.

ADDITIONAL PRENATAL TESTS FOR BABY:
- An ultrasound could be performed anytime during pregnancy — to verify the due date, look at the location of the placenta, or assess baby's growth or general well-being. If your pregnancy is going well and you're at low risk, an anatomy ultrasound may be your only one. But if you or baby have conditions that need extra supervision, more-frequent assessments may be done.
- A nonstress test (NST) involves placing monitors on mama's belly for about 20 minutes to assess fetal heart tones and uterine activity/contractions. It is typically done in the third trimester.
- A biophysical profile (BPP) combines an ultrasound and nonstress test to look at baby's heart rate, movement, muscle tone, breathing and amniotic fluid volume. A passing score gives a good sense of baby's general well-being.

#36

Coping with back pain: Part 2

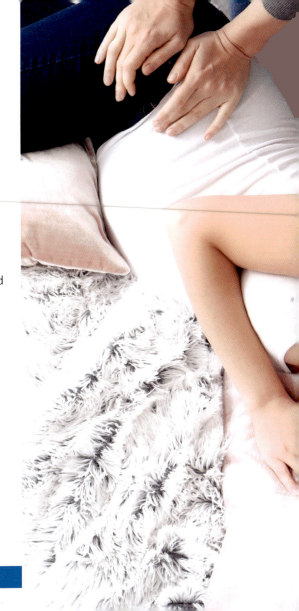

Here are some POSITIONS to try for back pain during labor:

- UPRIGHT — Stand, walk, slow dance, lunge. Side lunges are especially helpful, with your body and hips facing forward and your leg out to the side.
- LYING DOWN — Lie on your side or semiprone (on side but top shoulder and hip are rolled forward). Place pillows, a body pillow or a peanut-shaped ball in front of you with your leg resting on top to help open the pelvis.

- ALL FOURS — Lean forward (with or without ball) and do pelvic rocks.
- OPEN KNEE-CHEST POSITION — Get on all fours, knees spread comfortably apart, chest and head as low to the ground or bed as possible while hips remain high. Rest head on forearms or pillow.

#77

Prenatal tests and screenings

There is no test available with the result: "You have a perfect baby." However, please remember, the VAST majority of babies are born healthy overall.

INITIAL LAB WORK (early in pregnancy, ideally before 12 weeks):
· This analysis of blood and urine is to screen for infections, anemia and the presence of immunities, and to verify blood type.

ULTRASOUNDS:
· Anatomy (18 to 22 weeks) — Looks at all those precious baby parts! It also assesses the location of the placenta, just in case it's located near or over the cervix, which would require further follow-up. Baby's sex may also be revealed — if you so choose and if baby is cooperative.
· Additional ultrasounds may be done earlier or later in pregnancy. (See page 78.)

MIDPREGNANCY LABS:
· Glucose challenge test (24 to 28 weeks) — Screens moms for gestational diabetes after ingesting a sugary drink.
· Hemoglobin or complete blood count (CBC) — Checks for anemia.

GROUP B STREP, or GBS (35 to 37 weeks):
· A vaginal/rectal swab will be obtained to screen for bacteria called GBS. About 25% of women carry this bacteria and don't even realize it. If you test positive, your provider will recommend treatment with IV antibiotics while in labor to reduce the chance of transmission to baby. (See page 87 for more on this.)

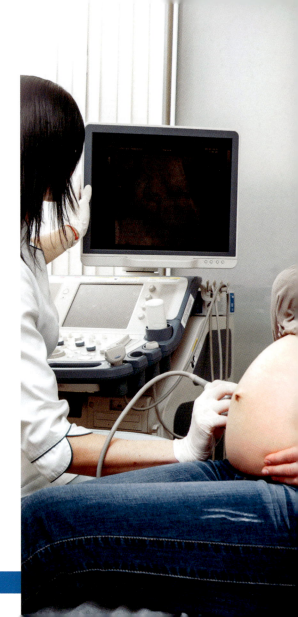

#37

Breathe

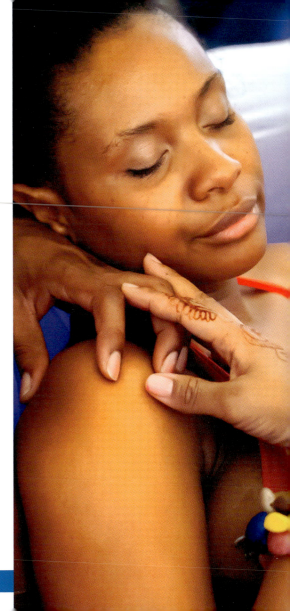

STEP 1: INHALE … (ENERGY, PEACE, STRENGTH)
STEP 2: EXHALE … (TENSION, STRESS, TIGHTNESS)

Anchor into this fact: Each breath is an extremely powerful tool. It can help you stay calm, relaxed and focused, release excess heat from your body, and lessen discomfort during contractions.

- Focus on DEEP BREATHING all the way down to expand your belly. This will provide oxygen to your baby and uterus, making for more-effective contractions. Try to do a slow count of at least four for each inhale and each exhale.
- CLEANSING BREATHS. Inhale through the nose. Exhale through the mouth.
- Keep your breathing sounds LOW VS. HIGH. Try it, and you'll feel the difference.

- At the END OF EVERY CONTRACTION, take another deep cleansing breath, adding an audible sigh. Exhale or moan to signal that the contraction is over, plus to release any residual tension.
- If slow, deep breaths aren't working anymore, change it up. The classic repetition of "HEE-HEE-HEE-HOO" throughout the contraction is an oldie but goody. This pattern of breathing may do the trick, especially later in the labor process.
- Let your INTUITION TAKE OVER, and you'll probably come up with your own variation. Go with it! The key is to keep the breaths happening with as much ease as possible.

#76

In case you're wondering

Certain topics — especially newer topics in the realm of pregnancy and parenting — can invite varied opinions and heated discussions. You may feel very strongly about the issues here, or maybe they weren't even on your radar yet. What do research and expert opinion say?

PLACENTOPHAGY:
- What it is: The practice of a woman consuming her placenta after birth. The placenta is often made into capsules but can be ingested in other forms too.
- The belief: It can help with milk supply, reduce postpartum depression and increase mom's iron stores.
- What current research says: There is no conclusive evidence that eating your placenta has benefits — and it could actually cause harm due to infections found in the placenta and the potential for contamination during processing.

VAGINAL SEEDING:
- What it is: Swabbing the mouth, nose or skin of a cesarean-born baby with gauze that was placed in the mom's vagina. This is done to inoculate the newborn with vaginal fluid that would naturally transfer bacteria during a vaginal birth.
- What is known: The microbiome — bacteria in the gut and on the body — of babies born by cesarean is initially different from that of babies born vaginally. Babies born by cesarean are more likely to have asthma, allergies, and immune and skin disorders. Is there a correlation?
- What current research says: By 6 months of age, the microbiomes of babies are the same, despite different modes of delivery. Since vaginal seeding could pass infections from mother to baby, the process isn't recommended unless part of a research study. But solid research says that

breastfeeding plays a big role in establishing a baby's microbiome — so nurse away!

MTHFR:
- What it is: A gene involved in how the body processes folate. With the rise of home DNA testing kits, some women are finding out that they have a variant of this gene. A quick internet search will reveal LOTS of discussion about it, including claims that a variant may cause neural tube defects (such as spina bifida) in a growing fetus or even recurrent early pregnancy loss.
- Currently: There is no change in folate/ folic acid recommendations based only on genetic test results. There's also no conclusive evidence to support screening for MTHFR variants, because they are highly prevalent and result in no change in care. And importantly, most women with MTHFR variants have normal, healthy pregnancies.

#38

End of labor phenomena (transition)

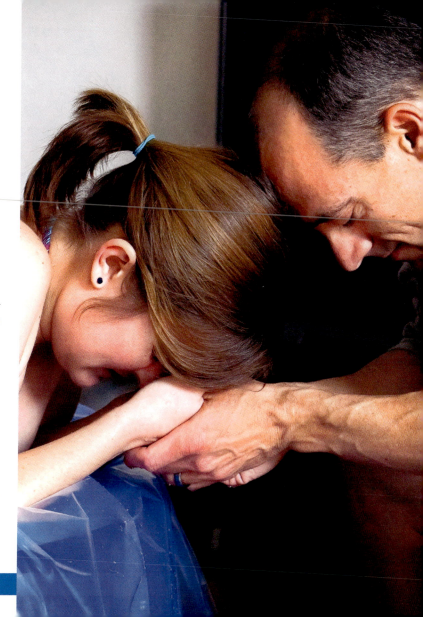

DON'T FREAK OUT

Toward the end of labor, also known as transition, your legs or whole body may tremble. You may feel nauseated and vomit (which typically brings relief from the nausea), feel cramps in your thighs and/or pressure in the pelvis, need to have a bowel movement, get very hot then cold, cry or cry out, want to give up, feel discouraged and frustrated, not want to be touched, or possibly withdraw into yourself. Hang in there! You're probably close to the end, as this part of labor is gearing up the body to push your baby out into the world.

- LABOR SUPPORT — Stay calm, close (make eye contact or keep your face near hers), and confident in her. Encourage her sweetly but with conviction.
- Transition may be followed by a SECOND WIND when mom becomes clearheaded, optimistic and determined. (You all deserve this!)
- AFTER TRANSITION some moms experience a pause in action when they may think things have regressed. This brief lull is a normal part of the process. Enjoy the calm and harness your energy because you'll be pushing soon!

#75

Intriguing research

NEW RESEARCH is always expanding our understanding of health in pregnancy and baby's first days. Here are a few areas in which scientists are making fascinating discoveries.

PREVENTING ALLERGIES AND ASTHMA:
- Studies show that the following may help prevent the development of allergies and asthma in children: Avoiding exposure to tobacco smoke, even while pregnant · consuming polyunsaturated fatty acids, especially omega-3, during pregnancy · having a full-term pregnancy · having a vaginal birth · breastfeeding exclusively for the first four to six months · reducing exposure to allergens (such as dust mites) · decreasing use of drying soaps and detergents · introducing solid foods gradually between four and six months of age, beginning with less allergenic foods (then eggs, dairy, peanuts, tree nuts, fish, shellfish)

CORD BLOOD:
- Cord blood is the blood that remains in the umbilical cord after the cord is clamped. It contains valuable stem cells that could help treat many different diseases, including some cancers.
- Unless you request otherwise, this potentially lifesaving blood will be discarded. Instead, parents can donate it to either a public cord blood bank or a research biobank, or they can pay to store it at a private cord blood bank to potentially use someday for their family. The American Academy of Pediatrics generally discourages private banking unless there is a family member who will benefit from it. Donating it is an opportunity to help others who are ill, or it could be used for research studies. Discuss options with your provider.

#39

Massage: Tips for the birth partner

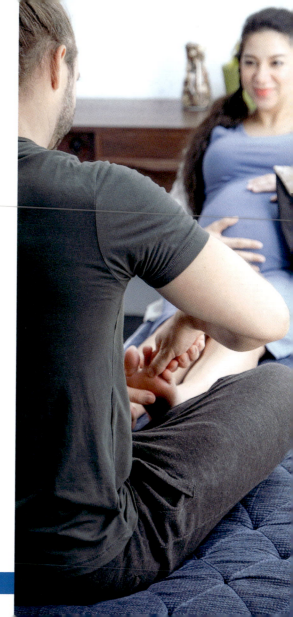

Ask mama to guide you ... and practice in advance for labor. These techniques typically feel great during pregnancy too. The typical bread-kneading approach may do the trick, but here are other methods to try:

- MASSAGE IN DOWNWARD MOTIONS in the direction of hair growth, which is calming and relaxing.
- GENTLY TRAIL YOUR HANDS down the lengths of the legs, starting from the hips down to the toes. Repeat over and over.
- PRETEND YOUR THUMBS are breaking a double ice pop (thumbs start together and glide outward), but do this technique on mom's hands/forearms/feet.
- DEEP, CIRCULAR massage with thumbs on the top side of the foot just below the ankle, 30 to 60 seconds at a time.
- CUP THE HEEL of the foot and squeeze as if you were squeezing a tennis ball. Release and repeat.

- Use a MASSAGE TOOL so that your hands won't get as tired.
- A small, FIRM BALL such as a lacrosse ball works great for self-massage too. Mama can roll a foot over the ball or press her back against the ball on a wall and roll around.
- Use MASSAGE OIL. Start with a small amount! Unscented may be preferred, as some aromas can become less than desirable for mom.
- You might be surprised by how much PRESSURE she likes during labor. Use one hand to support mom if the massage is pushing her forward.

#74

Postpartum mood changes

Bringing a baby home should provide for the most amazing, fulfilling and giddy feelings ever experienced ... right? Not always. Rapid hormone changes, exhaustion, doubt, lack of support, history of depression, unexpected birth outcomes and age can all contribute to postpartum blues, depression, anxiety or mood disorders. It's typically multifaceted. So what's normal, and when should you be concerned?

- BABY BLUES — Let's be honest, the first two weeks can be especially hard! During this timeframe, most women experience up-and-down emotions and feelings of being overwhelmed.
- POSTPARTUM MOOD DISORDER — If you have continued feelings of depression, anxiety, crying or irritability; feelings of hopelessness; difficulty in caring for yourself OR your baby or other children; feelings of wanting to hurt yourself or others; or difficulty in functioning, you may have postpartum depression. Approximately 10% to 15% of women experience this, along with many new fathers, and it can happen any time in the first year after a birth. Don't fight it alone. You're not being a bad parent, you're not going crazy and it's not your fault!

Try the following to manage your mental health:
- DAY TO DAY STEPS — Eat healthy. Get more sleep. Exercise. Get outside. Meditate or set aside time to relax. Practice mindfulness and/or spirituality. Minimize and declutter.
- DON'T ISOLATE — Talk to your partner, friends, family. You'll likely learn that you are not alone in this. If breastfeeding is taking too much of a toll, reevaluate.
- BEYOND SELF-CARE — Seek care with your OB provider or primary care provider. Your wellness is of the utmost importance — and your baby needs you! (Vibrant interactions with parents are important for babies' development!) Therapy and/or medications are often the KEYS for helping you cope during this time. There are safe medications you can take even if breastfeeding.
- RETURNING TO WORK — Take as much time off as you can to bond with baby and adjust to your new reality. If your employer can accommodate it, a gradual return to work (part time to full time) may help ease the transition.

#40

Double hip squeeze

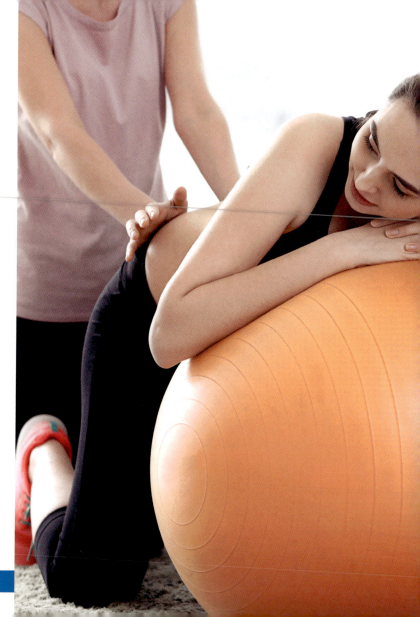

A TRIED-AND-TRUE MOVE TO HELP RELIEVE THE PRESSURE ON THE PELVIS DURING A CONTRACTION

- MOM — Lean forward against a wall or bed, or any variation of being on your hands and knees. Try gently swaying or rocking during contractions.
- BIRTH PARTNER — From behind mom, press her hips together, with your hands pushing toward each other. Apply steady pressure during contractions. Most women get the best relief from pressure at the top, flat part of the pelvis or lower down closer to the sacrum, though always rely on feedback from mom regarding the amount of pressure and best placement of palms on her buttocks/hips.
- VARIATIONS — If mom is on her hands and knees on the floor, her hips can be squeezed by the legs of someone standing/sitting behind her. Two-person option: Position someone on both sides of mama. (Note: This is most effective if both parties are pressing equally hard in the same area of both hips.)

#73

Breastfeeding benefits for mom

- LIKELY DECREASED RISK of breast cancer, uterine cancer, ovarian cancer, heart disease and type 2 diabetes.
- QUICKER POSTPARTUM RECOVERY — Baby's sucking helps the uterus shrink back to pre-pregnancy size faster and decreases the flow of postpartum bleeding and discharge (lochia), which means less blood loss. And producing all that milk burns up to 500 calories each day.
- MORE SLEEP! That's right — breastfeeding mamas actually get more zzz's and more restful sleep at night.
- COSTS LESS — Factor in the price of formula, bottles and supplies, even the potential of missed work and medical bills from additional illnesses — it adds up! There's a cost to the environment, too, for producing and distributing formula and supplies.

- No heating, sterilizing or mixing, which is ESPECIALLY HANDY at night.
- Nursing gives frequent opportunities for mama to REST and BOND with her baby.

IMPORTANT: Although breastfeeding is usually the best thing for mom and baby, there are times when donor milk or formula may be the best choice, or may even be medically necessary. The most important thing is for babies to be FED AND LOVED, and for mamas to be healthy and happy.

Note that DONOR MILK from a reliable milk bank has become the recommended alternative to breast milk, over formula, when supplementation is needed (according to leading breastfeeding organizations). But donor milk is typically more expensive and sometimes isn't a realistic option for families long-term. Donor milk or formula can be given by bottle, or by other methods that can help avoid nipple preference confusion if you're still trying to maintain a breasteeding relationship as well. Talk to a lactation specialist if you are wondering which feeding options are right for you, or if you have other questions about breastfeeding.

#41

Counterpressure

- During a contraction, apply STEADY and FIRM PRESSURE to an area of discomfort on mom (typically the low back, buttocks or tailbone).
- Use the PALM OR HEEL OF THE HAND as opposed to the fingers, which can be "pokey," for lack of a better word.
- As an alternative to the palm, make your hand into a FIST, and push the flat surface of your fingers against the low back. This keeps the wrist straight, protecting it from fatigue and discomfort. (Remove any large rings first.)
- Tennis balls or a massage tool might feel good, as well. Sometimes the best relief is A COLD SODA CAN right where it hurts. Put a couple on ice to have one ready when needed.
- Use one hand on the front of mom's hip to HELP BRACE HER while your other palm or fist is applying the counterpressure.

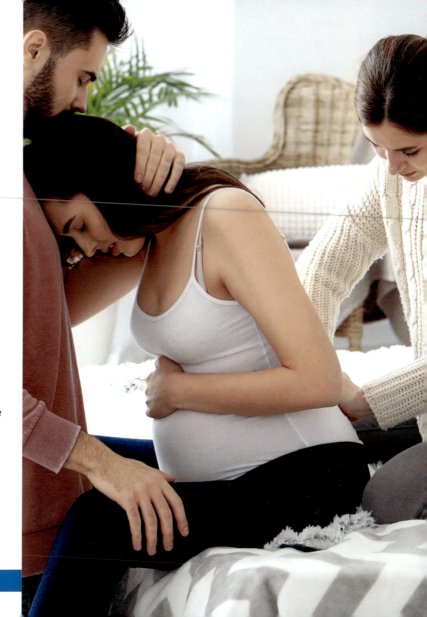

#72

Breastfeeding benefits for baby

Breastfeeding can be an incredible bonding time, but it can also be difficult. If you're looking for solid reasons to try breastfeeding or motivation to keep going, read on.

- Breastfeeding REDUCES THE RISK of sudden infant death syndrome (SIDS) and possibly childhood leukemia, according to some high-quality studies.
- It gives baby INFECTION-FIGHTING ANTIBODIES for immune defense. Formula-fed babies tend to have more colds, flu, ear infections, urinary tract infections and stomach problems.
- It enhances the development of HEALTHY BACTERIA in baby's digestive tract. Babies who don't get breast milk are more likely to develop allergies and asthma, juvenile diabetes, irritable bowel syndrome, rotavirus infection and high cholesterol.
- Breast milk contains 100+ INGREDIENTS not found in cow's milk that can't be synthesized in a laboratory for formula. Plus, it changes to meet baby's needs throughout the day and as baby grows.
- Breast milk is EASIER TO DIGEST for most babies. Cow's-milk-based and soy-based formulas can be hard on the newborn gut, causing excess gas, spitting up, constipation, and potential long-term digestive problems and food allergies.
- Breastfed babies have HEALTHIER SKIN with fewer skin conditions, such as eczema.
- Breastfeeding builds OPTIMAL ORAL DEVELOPMENT with proper alignment of baby's teeth, jaw, gums and palate and also fewer cavities.
- It leads to HEALTHY WEIGHT, with lower rates of obesity into toddlerhood, childhood and adulthood!
- The FATTY ACID DHA found in breast milk improves baby's vision and may even slightly increase a child's IQ.

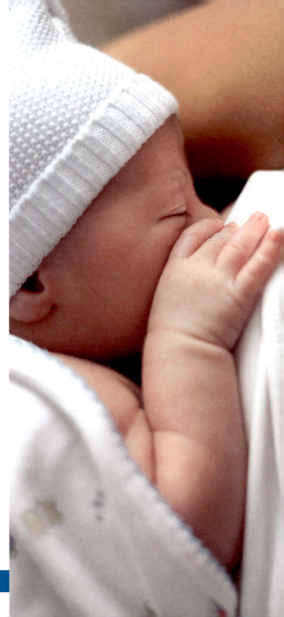

#42

Knowing what to say and when to say it

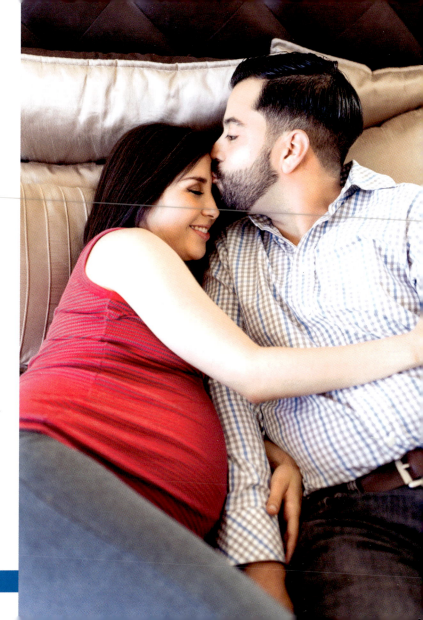

- HAVE PATIENCE and confidence in her — always. Trust your intuition as well, and ask care providers any questions you have ... but be supportive.
- Give her your UNDIVIDED ATTENTION.
- LISTEN to what she is saying. If she has worst-case thoughts, it might not be necessary to talk her out of them — she may need to get those out of her head in order to get the baby out of her body.
- GIVE UNSOLICITED PRAISE after every contraction. (Make your words mean something, though, or she may tune you out.)
- TAKE ONE CONTRACTION AT A TIME. "Just get through this one" might be a helpful reminder.
- DON'T ASK QUESTIONS DURING INTENSE CONTRACTIONS. You don't want to disrupt her rhythm or zone. She is probably in her more primitive brain, and if you ask her questions it will stimulate the neocortex part of her brain, which makes it harder to cope.
- MATCH HER MOOD, unless she needs encouragement or a distraction.
- PLEASE check your ego at the door and don't be offended by anything mama says or does.

#71

The animal in us all

If you forget everything else you learned about birth, remember this: Humans are animals, especially when having babies. So, what do you think happens when an animal in labor doesn't have her basics needs of survival (safety, food and water) met? Labor stops. The stress hormones that cause this reaction have a similar effect on people too — slowing contractions and potentially delaying labor. Stress hormones can also cause a heightened perception of pain (no thank you!). In addition, excessive levels of certain hormones decrease blood flow to the uterus and placenta, possibly causing distress to baby.

Here's the GOOD NEWS: This can be avoided if mama feels comfortable and can limit stress, fear and anxiety. Try the following:
- ASK for what you need to feel calm, safe, secure and well supported.
- BUILD A GOOD RELATIONSHIP with your care providers.
- PRACTICE the relaxation and coping tips throughout this book during pregnancy so your body is better trained to stay at ease.
- TAKE CHILDBIRTH EDUCATION CLASSES to build confidence with the process of birth and parenthood.
- Work with a DOULA.
- TOUR the hospital or birth center.
- CREATE THE BIRTH ENVIRONMENT you desire.
- EAT and DRINK throughout labor and birth if you're able.

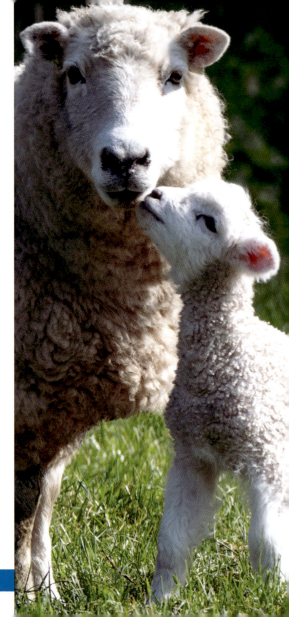

#43

The perineum

The perineum — the area between the vagina and the rectum — deserves a page in this book. It stretches and grows to accommodate baby's beautifully emerging head. The integrity and strength of the perineum during the process of birth can be affected by mom's health, genetics, length of pushing, mom's position and baby's position. Some of these factors you can control, some not. Here are several points to ponder or discuss with your medical provider.

- Consider doing PERINEAL MASSAGE at home starting at 36 weeks. Use a safe oil-based product to gently stretch and massage the perineal tissues just below the vagina. You can use your thumbs to provide this downward pressure. This helps prepare you to relax into the feeling of intense pressure in that same area on the day of your baby's birth.
- During the birth, have WARM COMPRESSES held to your perineum while pushing to reduce the risk of tearing.
- Listen for your PROVIDER'S CUES to help you guide baby out safely. Think of easing the baby out.

- AN EPISIOTOMY — a cut made in the perineum to widen the vaginal opening — used to be a common part of delivery. It's no longer done routinely because it can become infected, cause long-term pain and put mom at risk of a more significant tear. But episiotomies are sometimes medically necessary, such as when a faster delivery is needed due to concerns about baby's heart rate. Talk with your provider about his or her experience with episiotomies and your wishes.

#70

Hypnobirthing basics

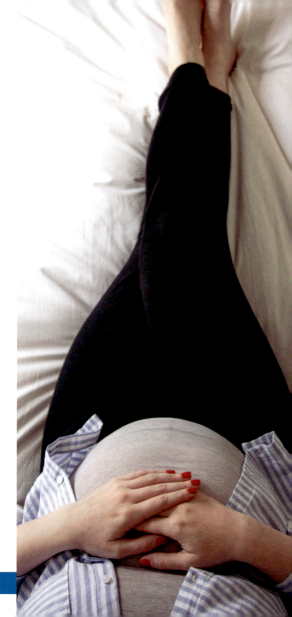

- WHAT — The premise of hypnobirthing is that creating calmness in the mind helps create relaxation in the body. Ideally, labor unfolds on its own timeline. Mom can have a state of mind similar to daydreaming to help the body do what it's meant to do, and birth can be peaceful, safe and satisfying.
- WHY — Self-hypnosis is a tool to promote deep relaxation for pregnancy, labor and birth, and even postpartum. All this could mean a better birth experience, less pain medication and quicker recovery with no known adverse effects. However, hypnotherapy may not be the right tool for women with a history of certain mental illnesses.
- WHEN — Any time fear enters the picture in labor, stress hormones are released, increasing heart rate and forcing blood to flow to the limbs (think fight-or-flight mode). That depletes blood flow to the uterus, potentially hindering labor. Relaxant hormones such as endorphins are what you want flowing!
- WHERE — Self-hypnosis can be done anywhere you can deeply relax. The more you practice, the more beneficial it tends to be.
- HOW — Try these steps:
  - Search online for classes near you and ask around for a personal referral.
  - Practice guided deep relaxation and breathing techniques. Self-hypnosis classes for birth typically offer resources to guide your practice.
  - Think or recite affirmations to feel empowered and trust in the birth process.
  - Verbalize and analyze fears or limiting thoughts to overcome them and let them go.

SO HELPFUL TO KNOW

#44

Let it go

There are some things about birth that your girlfriends — even the very best ones — don't share. Case in point: You might have a bowel movement when you push your baby out. Yep, sometimes it happens. As your baby moves down, he or she passes right past your bowels, so if something is there, it's going to come out. If that happens, it's a good sign to your care team — it means you are pushing well! The process may be over in one solid swoop, or it may happen bit by bit. Your nurse and provider are accustomed to such things and will be discreet. And your labor companion will just be proud of your hard work. So throw any shame or embarrassment aside, understand the normalcy, and focus on the task at hand: BIRTHING YOUR BABY!

Also of note: The same principle applies to urine.

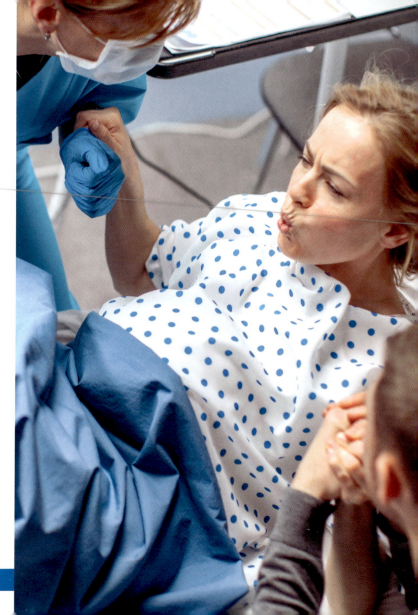

#69

Some essential essential oils

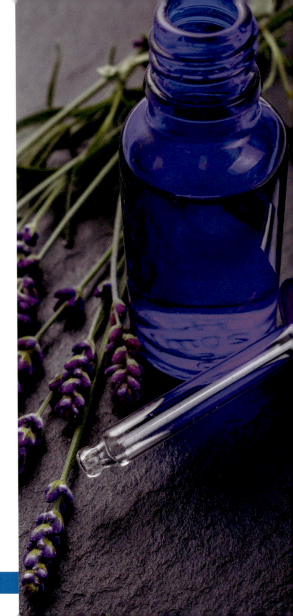

Essential oils have long been used for a variety of health-promoting benefits related to pregnancy and birth. With increasing scientific evidence, they are now finding their way into mainstream birth settings and hospitals. Hospitals may have restrictions on their use due to allergy concerns, so check ahead of time.

Depending on the brand and the oil, the oils may be smelled directly, diffused or applied to the skin. Ingesting oils during pregnancy is typically not recommended. When applied to the skin, most oils should be diluted in a carrier oil such as coconut oil or jojoba oil. Choose high-quality, pure oils.

Make sure to discuss any essential oils with your care provider before using during pregnancy. For use during labor, place a couple of drops on a tissue or cotton ball and store in a sealable container in case the aroma becomes less than desirable.

POPULAR OILS TO TRY:
- ANY CITRUS OIL such as lemon, orange or grapefruit — Can be very refreshing and energizing
- LAVENDER — Has calming and relaxing properties, promotes restful sleep
- SPEARMINT or PEPPERMINT — May help ease digestive issues and upset stomach, manage headaches, clear nasal congestion and improve focus
- GINGER — May help with occasional nausea or indigestion during pregnancy and during transition in labor

If your hospital offers essential oils for use during labor, you can just ask to try theirs.

#45

Time to push

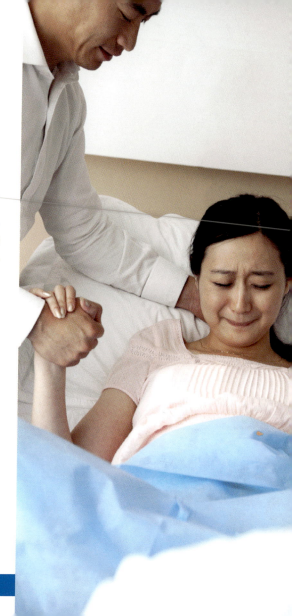

- THE URGE TO PUSH often coincides with full dilation. You'll feel pressure or the need to have a bowel movement.
- MOM'S POSITION while pushing should vary. Try upright (including standing, kneeling, squatting or using a birthing stool), hands-and-knees, side-lying or semireclined positions. An epidural or baby's heart rate may limit certain positions. Being upright may allow gravity to help baby down the birth canal. Research shows that it may shorten the pushing phase and even help avoid an episiotomy and the use of forceps or vacuum assistance. Lying on your side may lead to less tearing. Pushing while on your back or semireclined may not be as effective because of the angle of the pelvis and the constriction that the bed puts on your tailbone area. Your medical provider or a nurse can watch closely and let you know what's working.

- RELEASE/RELAX the pelvic floor and your bottom. Think of a bulge in your pelvis, and let it be heavy instead of trying to hold it in.
- Pushing when you have SPONTANEOUS URGES maximizes your body's natural reflexes.
- You may feel baby losing ground between contractions — that's OK! Baby's descent can be THREE STEPS FORWARD, TWO STEPS BACK, helping baby's head adjust to the pressure and stretch the perineum.
- THE CROWNING MOMENT — As baby's head crowns, you may feel intense burning or the "ring of fire." Stop pushing and blow lightly with chin lifted. Listen to your provider for direction — this may help minimize tearing. Reach down and feel baby's head!
- Before those last pushes, GET READY! Have the designated person grab the camera if you want to capture baby's arrival!

PUSHING

#68

Acupressure

Acupressure is an ancient technique of applying pressure to certain points on the body to help balance the flow of chi — loosely translated as vital energy or life force. Here are several traditional acupressure points that may help reduce labor pain and potentially speed up labor too.

Note: These techniques should be discussed with your care provider and should not be done prior to 39 weeks, as they may have some potential for inducing labor prematurely. More research is needed on this possible effect.

ACUPRESSURE 101:
- Press firmly into the acupressure point with a thumb, a knuckle, or a blunt object like a pen or the eraser-end of a pencil.
- The spot will feel slightly more tender than the surrounding area.
- Press for 30 seconds, release for 10 seconds; repeat for a total of five minutes or longer, if desired.
- Continually take slow, deep, cleansing breaths.
- Locations to try:
  - LARGE INTESTINE 4 — It can alleviate pain and possibly regulate contractions. Press on the back of the hand, in the webbing between the thumb and index finger near where the bones come together.
  - SPLEEN 6 — Try here to help regulate contractions and dilate the cervix. About four finger-widths above the inside of the ankle bone, press into the side of the shin bone.
- BLADDER 67 — This position may promote fetal movement and may help babies get into a more optimal position for birth. Press into the outside lower corner of the nail of the little toe.
- LIVER 3 — Thought to relieve stress and soften the cervix, this point is one finger-width below the area between the base of the big toe and second toe.
- BLADDER 60 — This point may help ease labor pain and encourage better fetal positioning. Press in the space between your ankle bone and Achilles tendon.

#46

Comfort measures while pushing

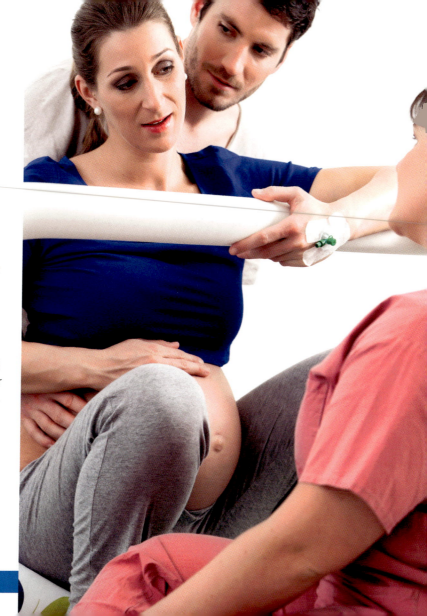

- PARTNER — Help mom stay balanced in whatever position she chooses and give her support. She may need a person to lean into or want you to lend support to a leg.
- MOM — Relax your face, especially your jaw and mouth, because it helps relax your upper (and lower!) body, focusing all energy to an effective push. Take cues from your provider or nurse — he or she can give you feedback about how you're pushing and what pushes are most effective.
- CHANGE POSITIONS every 20 to 30 minutes or so if progress seems to have plateaued. Options include squatting, kneeling on all fours, standing, lying on your side and sitting semireclined. Ask your nurse or provider for tools, such as a birthing stool or a birthing bar.
- You may want A MIRROR to be able to see baby's grand debut! Don't worry if you see wrinkles and a gray-blue skin color on baby. These are typical side effects of traveling through the birth canal.
- Have specific MUSIC PLAYING, if you'd like.

#67

TOLAC/VBAC

You may be familiar with the term *VBAC*, or vaginal birth after cesarean. So why is your doctor or midwife talking about a TOLAC? A birth isn't a successful VBAC until you've actually HAD the vaginal birth. Prior to that, you are considered a candidate (or not) for trial of labor after cesarean (TOLAC). After having one cesarean birth, many women are faced with the decision of choosing a repeat cesarean or attempting a TOLAC with their next child.

Points to discuss with your medical provider:

- AVAILABILITY — Does your hospital or medical provider offer TOLACs? Not all do.
- CHANCE OF SUCCESS — Your provider will look at your age, BMI and other factors that affect the chance of a successful VBAC.
- WHY THE CESAREAN WAS DONE — Providers consider whether the reason for your previous cesarean is likely to repeat. If your cesarean was done because of fetal heart rate concerns when you were 7 cm dilated, that may not happen again. It's more concerning if you had a cesarean because you pushed for four hours and the baby never descended low into the pelvis. That scenario could repeat.
- UTERINE INCISION FROM YOUR CESAREAN — If there was an extension of the incision higher up on your uterus or it was vertical, versus low transverse or horizontal, it won't be safe for you to attempt TOLAC. The risk of an incision opening is much higher.
- SAFETY AND RECOVERY — Vaginal birth is typically safer than a cesarean, and recovery is quicker and easier. However, discuss your personal circumstances.
- RISK OF UTERINE RUPTURE — The old uterine incision could open during labor, although for most women the risk of this is <1%.
- YOUR DESIRED FAMILY SIZE — If your goal is to have several children, it's safest to avoid multiple cesareans because risks increase with each one.

If you're interested in TOLAC, maximize your chances!

- Start your pregnancy at a healthy weight and stay within the recommended weight gain.
- Choose a medical provider whose thoughts align with yours and who supports TOLAC.
- Ideally, space your pregnancies by 18 months or longer.
- Read up on normal labor and vaginal birth, and allow for spontaneous labor rather than induced labor, if possible.
- Surround yourself with good labor support (partner, doula, another trusted person).

#47

Bond, nurse, marvel, fall in love!

- IMMEDIATE SKIN-TO-SKIN CONTACT! This releases hormones that benefit you and baby. Oxytocin promotes bonding and helps the uterus contract down to its normal size. Endorphins help make you calm and responsive to your baby. Your little bundle will be toweled off to help prevent him or her from getting chilled. Your body warms the baby, so keep that bundle close without clothing other than a diaper in between. (You can cover both of you with a blanket.) Skin-to-skin time may help stabilize baby's heart rate. Other possible benefits include increased immunity, improved attention, less crying, and a lower risk of colic and sleep disorders.
- HAT — It's cute, but may not be needed unless baby is preterm or has a lower birth weight or baby's temperature is a concern. Research suggests that the smell of baby's head may actually help trigger an elaborate hormonal response in mom that benefits both.
- Allow baby plenty of uninterrupted time to begin to nurse, which can take up to an hour or so. This STRONGLY INFLUENCES MILK PRODUCTION and is best done by allowing baby to lead the way. (Avoid the "smash and grab" technique.) Good things can take time.
- Baby will typically be VERY ALERT FOR ONE TO TWO HOURS after birth, called the golden hour. So take that time to get to know your baby — usually, everything else can wait.

- HOLDING BABE TO CHEST is a wonderful way to help him or her transition from the womb. Baby can still smell your scent and hear your heartbeat and familiar voice. Give baby skin-to-skin time with the birth partner, too, as there are similar benefits. Research supports doing this intermittently during these first weeks.
- Don't forget to snap some PHOTOS in those first moments of life. It's hard to know what you'll remember or wish you had documented, especially if you're exhausted from labor! Better yet — hand that CAMERA to your nurse or doula to capture those incredible first images of your family.
- Invite VISITORS ONLY WHEN YOU'RE READY — You deserve to savor the precious, intimate early time with baby. Typically, it's best to limit visitors for the first 24 to 48 hours to allow you time to rest, heal and get feeding off to the best start possible. You only get this time once!
- ROOMING IN — Long gone are the days of healthy babies spending hours in the hospital nursery away from their parents. Take these first days to learn the sounds and cues of your baby. Newborns need to feed frequently, and the frequent stimulation will help mom to establish a good milk supply. Mom may even sleep better at night when babe is rooming in.

#66

Water birth 101

Many mamas find water to be an effective pain reliever when laboring and want to take this through birth. If you're interested in having your baby emerge into this world from the water, the basics are covered here.

It's important to know that the safety of water birth is still debated among groups of experts. The American College of Obstetricians and Gynecologists advises against pushing and delivering in the water, due to limited data on the benefits versus the risks. The American Academy of Pediatrics also advises against it. Meanwhile, the American College of Nurse-Midwives supports water birth as an option for uncomplicated pregnancies if it's a parent's informed, shared decision with a medical provider.

Talk with your doctor or midwife about the following:
- RISKS and BENEFITS — There have been rare cases of breathing in water (aspiration), umbilical cord snap and infection among babies born in the water. Benefits may include higher satisfaction with birth, less pain, less use of pain medications, possibly shorter labor and less need for an episiotomy.
- AVAILABILITY — Is it possible where you're birthing? Do providers at the facility offer it? How many tubs are there, and what type of tub do they have?
- CRITERIA — What are the requirements, including tests, procedures and protocols, to make water birth possible?
- EXCLUSIONS — What situations might come up in pregnancy, labor or birth that would make it necessary for the birth to take place out of the water? In those cases, is laboring in the tub still an option?
- TIMING — Providers have different opinions about the "best" time to use hydrotherapy, so be sure to ask yours when you can hop in.

#48

Procedures for mom

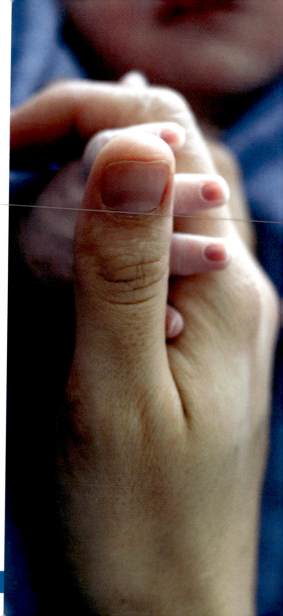

Baby's out, but there are a few more things left to do for mom. The good news is that you can most likely hold and nurse your babe the whole time.

- THE UMBILICAL CORD will continue to pulsate after baby is born, delivering extra blood (including millions of stem cells) that would have otherwise remained in the placenta. This extra boost helps with baby's iron stores, which may have long-term benefits for health and development. The recommended delay for cord clamping is at least 30 to 60 seconds for full-term babies. Cord clamping may potentially be delayed up to three to five minutes to deliver additional blood. If desired, someone can have the honor of cutting the cord once your provider clamps it. Mamas: Feel free to take on this task yourself.
- THE PLACENTA will detach from the uterus and be expelled, usually within five to 30 minutes of birth, known as the third stage of labor. You may feel cramping, mild contractions or fullness in your vagina. Additional pushing efforts may be required to birth the placenta, but remember that it's soft and nothing like a baby coming out! If you're curious, ask to see this amazing organ that nourished your growing baby.
- Your CARE PROVIDER WILL ASSESS the perineum, vagina and vulva for any tearing, and will repair the perineal area if needed using a local anesthetic and dissolvable stitches.
- In the minutes and hours after birth, the nurse and care provider will also monitor any bleeding from mom and how well the UTERUS IS CONTRACTING to return to a healthy, firm state. This will be done with uterine massage and/or certain medications.

#65

Pregnancy sleep tips

Being pregnant is exhausting! And yet, just when you need rest the most, your slumber may be interrupted by needing to go to the bathroom, restless legs, sudden leg cramps and an inability to get comfortable. The not-so-dreamy hormones and changes to your body can even cause snoring or sleep apnea. You deserve a solid night's rest, so try these tips:

- DARKNESS — The brain may interpret any trace of light as a signal to wake up, so sleep in complete darkness. The simplest way to do this is to wear an eye mask. When you need to get up to use the bathroom, keep the lights dim.
- EARLY BEDTIME — Your pregnant body NEEDS sleep. Feel like you need an excuse to crash early? Your body knows sleep is its prime time to repair and recharge.
- LIMIT EVENING LIQUIDS — To decrease the nighttime need to go to the bathroom, curb your liquid intake the last couple of hours before you go to bed.
- BEDTIME SNACKS — When reaching for those "last call" foods, opt for protein and healthful fats rather than foods high in sugar. Protein can provide l-tryptophan to produce melatonin and serotonin, which help regulate sleep. Conversely, elevated blood sugar inhibits sleep.

- TEMPERATURE — Below 70 degrees Fahrenheit is ideal to be comfortably cool.
- UNPLUG — The light emitted from cellphones, computers and TVs — along with the content you read or watch — can stimulate the brain. Try eliminating screens an hour or so before bed. Overnight, silence or turn off phones when possible. Ideally, keep electronics (including alarm clocks) away from your bed to avoid the light and noise they may give off.
- PILLOWS — When lying on your side, you may appreciate having several extra pillows (under your abdomen, between your knees and behind you). Upgrading to a long or U-shaped body pillow may be just what you need to get cozy.
- RELAX — Practice the relaxation techniques on page 24, and sprinkle in rituals such as aromatherapy, massage or a bath to unwind.

#49

The look of a typical newborn

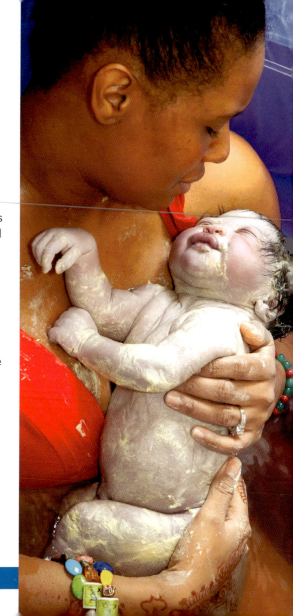

- BLUISH SKIN — As circulation begins, baby's bluish coloring will fade, but the hands and feet sometimes remain blue for the first few hours.
- VERNIX — This thick, sticky cream protected your baby from the amniotic fluid in the womb and continues to protect him or her on the outside. It's full of antibacterial and antimicrobial properties, so let it fully absorb into baby's skin for at least 24 hours before giving a bath.
- MISSHAPEN HEAD — Most babies have an oblong, cone-shaped head from time spent in the birth canal, possibly with swelling and/or bruising. Hey, it's tough to be born. Don't worry, the head WILL mold back into a nice, round shape within a few days.
- MILIA — These little whitehead-looking spots will disappear within a few weeks.

- SWOLLEN BREASTS OR GENITALS — This swelling is due to mom's hormones and will not even be noticeable within a few days.
- LANUGO — This fine, possibly dark hair may cover the body and will be shed in the weeks after birth.
- RED PATCHES — Sometimes babies are born with "stork bites" or red patches, commonly on the back of the neck or on the face. These are temporary and will fade over the upcoming weeks or months.
- OTHER — Whenever you have questions about what's normal or not normal as you discover every inch of your newborn, ask your nurse or baby's medical provider.

#64

Post-birth

- PHYSICAL ASPECTS — Delivery of placenta (five to 30 minutes or so after birth) · uterine massage · repair any tears, if needed
- EMOTIONAL ASPECTS — Relief · pride · joy · exhilaration · increased energy followed by exhaustion
- WHAT MAMA SHOULD DO — Hold baby skin to skin · give baby opportunities to latch on · talk to and admire baby · breathe to cope with any discomfort · after some much-deserved cuddle time, allow baby to be weighed and examined as needed — most other procedures for the baby can wait (see page 50)
- WHAT LABOR PARTNER SHOULD DO — Take pictures and video · cut umbilical cord, if desired · enjoy skin-to-skin contact with baby · go with the baby, if separation is necessary

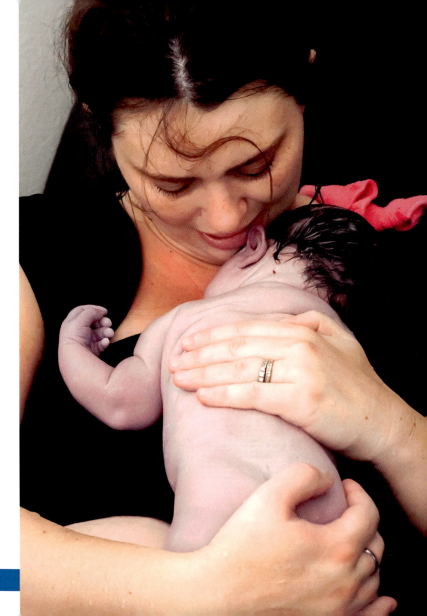

#50

Procedures for baby

- APGAR SCORE — This is a snapshot of how well baby is doing as he or she transitions to life outside the womb. The score is checked at 1 and 5 minutes of age, assessing color, muscle tone, heart rate, breathing and reflexes. This test is done visually, often with baby on your chest.
- VITAMIN K INJECTION — This is given in baby's thigh to help promote healthy blood clotting. It's important but can easily be delayed until after your first nursing session or possibly even while nursing, so baby will barely notice.
- ANTIBIOTIC OINTMENT — This ointment is put on the eyes, mainly to prevent the transmission of gonorrhea and chlamydia. This can also be delayed in order for your baby to get a good look at you without extra cloudiness in his or her eyes.
- MEASUREMENTS — Get the specs on that new baby! Length and weight will be recorded soon after birth. However, this doesn't need to happen immediately. It's OK to make skin-to-skin contact your #1 priority before getting those measurements. (You probably won't be sending out birth announcements in the first hour anyway!)

- HEPATITIS B VACCINE — The first dose of three doses is recommended in the hospital. Talk to your baby's provider if you have any questions about the timing of vaccinations.
- CIRCUMCISION for boys — If this is desired, make sure to do your research, including checking insurance coverage, ahead of time and ask your care team any questions. For hospital births, circumcision is often performed during the hospital stay.
- OTHER POSSIBLE TESTS — Before heading home, baby may have bilirubin levels tested to check for jaundice, one more weight check, and screenings for metabolic disorders, early hearing loss, and/or some congenital cardiac defects. If you return home the same day from a birth center, these may happen at a follow-up visit within the first few days.

Talk with your care provider, baby's provider or hospital staff if you have any questions about newborn procedures and recommendations. Also know that you can most likely stay with your baby during any procedures.

#63

Pushing

- PHYSICAL ASPECTS — Urge to push · intense pelvic pressure · temporary break from contractions
- EMOTIONAL ASPECTS — Excitement · anxiety · focus · renewed energy
- WHAT MAMA SHOULD DO — Bear down with natural urges · relax pelvic floor · change positions as needed
- WHAT LABOR SUPPORT SHOULD DO — Support mom's instinctive positions · guide her if needed · have the camera nearby · give visualizing cues, such as saying, "down your spine and out your body"

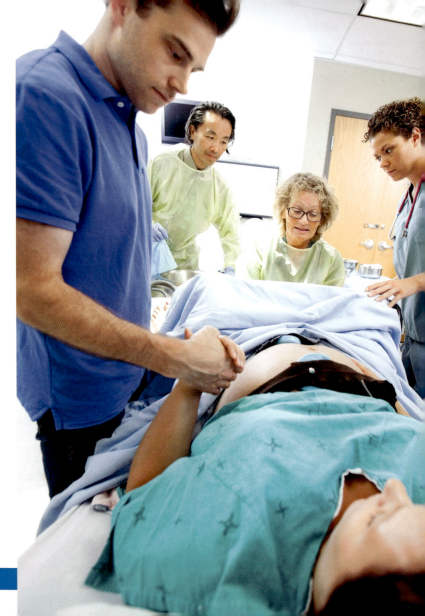

#51

Breastfeeding secrets worth sharing

While breastfeeding is an instinctual process, there's definitely a learning curve. Keep these things in mind as you get started:

- LAID-BACK BREASTFEEDING — You can try having baby on your chest, leading the way; you recline enough to let gravity hold the baby, relaxed and comfortable.
- ANTICIPATE — Better to watch your baby, not the clock. It's easiest to feed before babe gets "hangry." Hunger cues could be rooting — opening the mouth and turning the head to suck — tongue sucking, moving hand to mouth or making noises.
- LATCH — Touch your nipple on baby's upper lip to stimulate baby to open his or her mouth. Get baby to open wide to take in more of the breast, not just the nipple. A deep latch will reduce nipple soreness AND help baby get milk efficiently. If you need to reposition, gently slip your clean finger into baby's mouth to release the latch.
- BABY'S ALIGNMENT — Baby is in a good position if the ear, shoulder and hip are in a straight line. Try this: Turn your own head to the right or left and swallow. Not easy, right?
- CHECK — Baby's mouth should be wide open with lips flanged (think fish lips). The first few days the swallows will be small and spaced out, but make sure you are comfortable identifying what a swallow looks and sounds like before you take baby home.

- TIME — Don't rush the process. Breastfeeding isn't fast food, but it'll become efficient. Use the help available while in the hospital or birth center to get your best start.
- SUPPORT — Find other breastfeeding mamas to share wisdom, and seek help from an International Board Certified Lactation Consultant (IBCLC) if you need it. Nipple tenderness can be normal the first few days during the initial 10 to 30 sucks. But call a lactation specialist if you have pain beyond that or notice damage to the nipple. NOTE: If breastfeeding continues to be painful or a struggle, have baby's provider double-check that your babe isn't tongue-tied or lip-tied (short frenulum), which could hinder a proper latch.
- GOOD MILK SUPPLY — Frequent feedings and emptying the breasts are key. Alternate which side you offer first. Let baby feed until done on the first side, then offer the second side. If baby is full, just start on that fuller breast with the next feeding.
- HYDRATION — Mom needs to stay hydrated too! Many women feel parched when breastfeeding, so keep water within reach.
- BODY MECHANICS — Gather those props. Use pillows to help support your arms and bring baby close to your breast, rather than you leaning forward. Propping your feet up on a footstool may be more comfortable, too.

#62

Transition

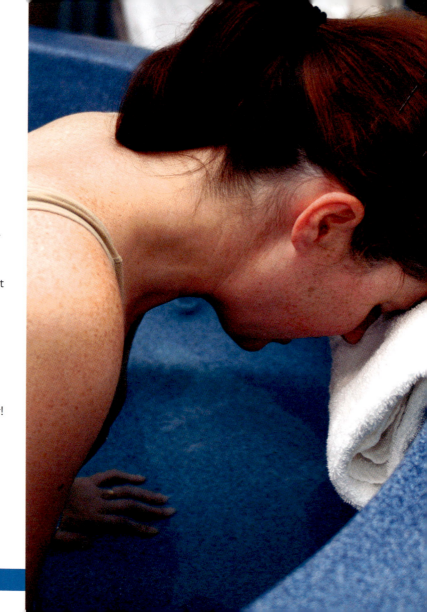

- PHYSICAL ASPECTS — Hot/cold flashes · shaking/trembling · nausea (possibly with vomiting) · intense and close contractions · typically the shortest phase, lasting minutes to two hours · cervix opens from 7 to 10 cm on average
- EMOTIONAL ASPECTS — Anticipation · loss of focus · self-doubt · intense anxiety
- WHAT MAMA SHOULD DO — Keep breathing · dig deep and remember how strong you are · take one contraction at a time, or even half of a contraction at a time (the second half gets easier since it's after the peak) · eat small bites and take sips of fluids if allowed · if the urge to push is overbearing but it's just not time, take short breaths while you say "pa-pa-pa" until the urge passes · remember that often, just when you can't take it anymore, it's over!
- WHAT LABOR SUPPORT SHOULD DO — Stay close · remain calm, confident and kind · help mom maintain focus (If she says she can't do this, tell her in an encouraging way, "You ARE doing this!") · acknowledge the difficulty, but remind her that baby will be in her arms soon!

#52

Heal thyself

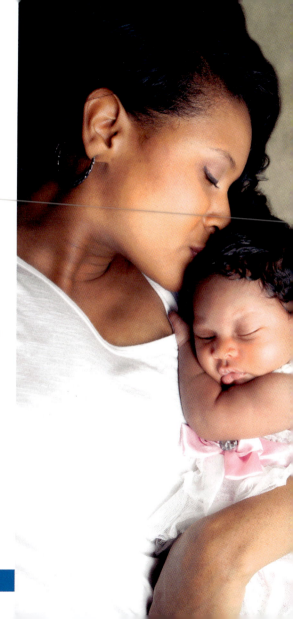

- Line up WITCH HAZEL PADS on a feminine pad to soothe the area of baby's grand entrance. These are also helpful if hemorrhoids are an issue.
- Meet your new best friend: THE PERI BOTTLE. Fill this little squirt bottle with warm water and squirt on the perineum while you're urinating to help relieve any stinging. This also provides a gentle way to wash afterward. Then gently pat dry.
- COLD PACKS on the perineum after birth are "Amazing" with a capital A for calming inflammation, especially in the first 24 hours.
- Keep those STOOLS LOOSE — You may opt to take a stool softener or natural senna laxative, but also drink plenty of water and eat enough fiber.
- And when it comes to those first post-birth bowel movements, you may find that using some of your LABOR RELAXATION TECHNIQUES and/or breathing is helpful.
- Soak your bottom in WARM WATER for 20 minutes, three times a day. This could be in your bathtub or in a special bowl (sitz bath) found in most drugstores. The warmth helps promote healing and feels fabulous — great with or without special postpartum herbs.
- KEGEL EXERCISES can stimulate circulation that will help with healing. Do them more gently than during pregnancy, to start. You may not feel like you're activating those muscles, but keep trying — perhaps when you nurse your sweet babe.
- AVOID THE PHYSICAL DEMANDS OF LIFTING heavy objects or prolonged sitting or standing until you feel recovered, which is typically four to six weeks.

#61

Active labor

- PHYSICAL ASPECTS — Contractions become longer, stronger and closer together · increased bloody show · cervix is likely dilated 5 to 6 cm and typically continues opening 1 cm every one to two hours until pushing
- EMOTIONAL ASPECTS — Less talkative between contractions · increased focus
- WHAT MAMA SHOULD DO — Try various comfort measures · perform slow/deep breathing · try rhythmic rituals to cope with contractions · eat and drink if allowed (think small bites and sips as opposed to a full meal) · suck on ice chips · relax · change positions periodically
- WHAT LABOR SUPPORT SHOULD DO — Drive mom to the hospital or birth center if you're not there already · help her rest between contractions · remind her to relax (face, shoulders, other areas) · suggest positions · offer comfort measures

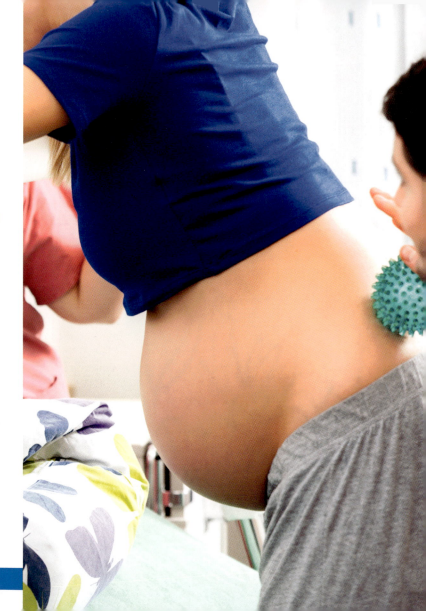

#53

Rest

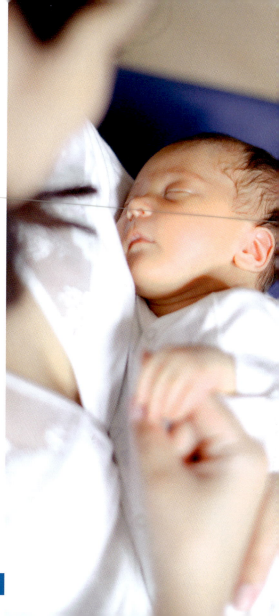

ACT LIKE YOU JUST HAD A BABY!

Newborns typically sleep up to 16 or 17 hours a day, so take advantage of this time to recover.

- In order for your pelvic floor muscles to have the BEST AND FASTEST RECOVERY and to minimize postpartum bleeding, give yourself permission to be horizontal and rest more than usual — especially those first two weeks.
- Initially, growing babies need to eat up to 10 OR MORE TIMES IN 24 HOURS. This new (and temporary) schedule can be a difficult adjustment. Feeding a newborn can feel overwhelming, no matter whether you're nursing, pumping or formula-feeding. Babies start to space feedings out more over time, but it is a real commitment. Try to enjoy those quiet moments with baby and remind yourself that things will get easier. Try napping throughout the day to make up for lost sleep at night — that whole "sleep when baby sleeps" is a REAL thing.
- GETTING ADEQUATE REST will help prevent postpartum depression and ease the transition into your family's new reality.
- GET HELP with meals, laundry and household chores. It really does take a village to raise a baby!
- Many cultures have customs for built-in SUPPORT. The new mama may be mentored by more experienced mothers; get help for a while with older children, meals and tasks; or even stay with grandparents to help ease the transition to parenthood. So please, at least entertain the idea of not entertaining.

#60

Early labor

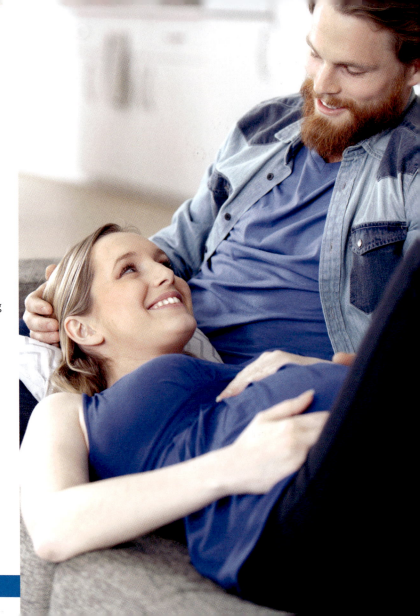

- PHYSICAL ASPECTS — Contractions in a pattern (getting longer, stronger and closer together) · bloody show (possibly) · cervix opens to 5 to 6 cm on average, which may take hours to days
- EMOTIONAL ASPECTS — Uncertainty · talkative between contractions · excitement
- WHAT MAMA SHOULD DO — Relax · practice slow, deep breathing · alternate between rest and activity · take a bath or shower · apply ice or heat if experiencing low backache · eat and drink
- WHAT LABOR SUPPORT SHOULD DO — Offer massage · time contractions periodically · contact other labor support · provide distraction (games, TV, a walk and so on)

#54

Read the baby, not just the book

Your baby doesn't come with an owner's manual, and for good reason. You will write the book on your baby by doing the following:

- WATCH — Right from birth, babies provide cues as to when they are hungry, tired or soiled.
- LISTEN — Crying can mean many different things, and as time goes by you'll learn whether it means hungry, tired, overstimulated or bored, and everything in between. Providing a quick response to babies' cries teaches them they can trust the world.
- RELAX — Babies pick up on others' energy, so a relaxed parent breeds a relaxed child, and vice versa. (Temporarily — although relaxing is a good long-term life skill to practice.)
- BE PATIENT — All babies are transitioning to life on the outside of the womb. For some, this can take three to four months or more. Remember: Enjoy the joys, and the challenging stages shall pass!

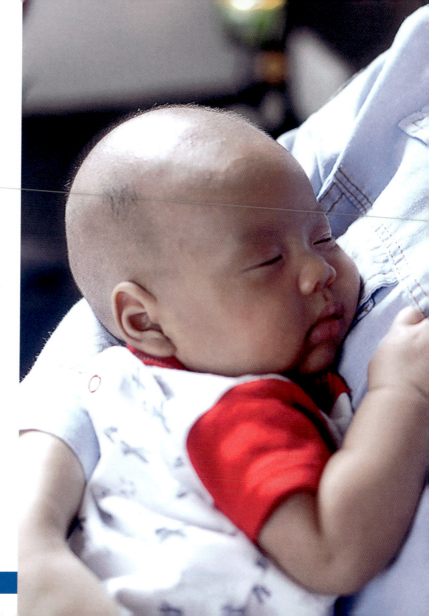

#59

Prelabor

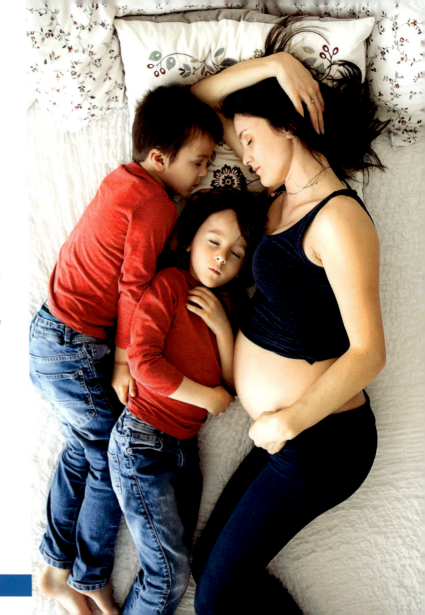

- PHYSICAL ASPECTS — Two to four weeks before birth: nesting · low back pain · frequent/loose stools · loss of mucous plug · increase in Braxton Hicks contractions · lightening or tummy "dropping" (making breathing easier but increasing vaginal zingers — when you feel them, you'll know it)
- EMOTIONAL ASPECTS — Nervousness · anxiety · impatience
- WHAT MAMA SHOULD DO — Rest in preparation for birth · take walks · do deep breathing · complete final preparations · enjoy the last "pre-baby" days
- WHAT LABOR SUPPORT SHOULD DO — Have fun with mom · keep her from overdoing it

#55

Ensuring adequate nutrition for babe

Monitoring baby's weight gain is something your pediatrician or care provider will help you do, which is why those INITIAL CHECK-UPS ARE SO IMPORTANT.

Paying attention to diapers will help you know if your baby's getting enough nutrition. By the time your newborn is 4 to 5 days old, he or she should typically have six to eight WET DIAPERS each day. Expect babe to want to eat eight to 12 times a day or more. (Remember: Baby's stomach is only about the size of his or her tiny fist!)

Also, KEEPING A RECORD of baby's daily feedings and diaper details on a tracking sheet or app can really help get everyone on a healthy path. Ask for a form where you deliver, or find a smartphone tracking app.

THE SCOOP ON POOP — Baby's first stools, called meconium, are thick, sticky and tarlike. After this meconium has passed, breastfed babies' stools will transition to a soft, seedy and mustard-yellow color. Formula-fed babies' stools have more of a thick pudding consistency, yellow or brown in color.

Most babies will tolerate MOM'S DIET without issue. But sometimes baby's digestive system may not be quite ready. Contact your provider if baby develops a rash, excessive fussiness, gas or a chronic runny nose. Adjusting mom's diet until baby's gastrointestinal (GI) tract further develops may do the trick, so evaluate potential dietary changes with your baby's provider. Also ask him or her about VITAMIN D SUPPLEMENTS for baby, especially if you're breastfeeding.

Note: If you're breastfeeding, the American Academy of Pediatrics suggests holding off from using a pacifier for three to four weeks, until nursing is well established. It could interfere with breastfeeding, as some babies may have a hard time with the differences between sucking while nursing and pacifier sucking. Pacifier sucking also may unintentionally delay a feeding. New babies need to eat often, and pacifier use too early or too often may affect the supply and demand of milk production.

#58

Overview of labor

- PRELABOR — The cervix may begin the opening process with a combination of softening, thinning (effacing) and some opening (dilating), along with moving forward to align with the birth canal (vagina). Mild, erratic contractions may occur but may go totally unnoticed. Baby begins the process of descent and rotation to make his or her way out.
- EARLY LABOR — The cervix continues to soften and efface and begins dilating more. Start using rituals for contractions to try to stay relaxed. Have patience with early labor, as it can last for several hours (or one or more days).
- ACTIVE LABOR — Here, contractions are intensifying and are more consistent, causing the cervix to change. Especially use the hands-on tricks on pages 25 and 39-41.
- TRANSITION — The cervix dilates to the full 10 centimeters (cm). Baby descends more into the birth canal. Contractions are very close together and intense.
- PUSHING — This is the last stretch of the marathon. With pushing efforts, baby makes the final descent and rotates his/her head. Listen closely to your body, support team and care provider to guide you through the birthing process. Pushing and birthing your baby can potentially last several minutes or several hours. It's typically longer for first-time mothers and quicker for those who have had a vaginal birth before.
- POST-BIRTH — Delivery of the placenta usually occurs within five to 30 minutes of birth.

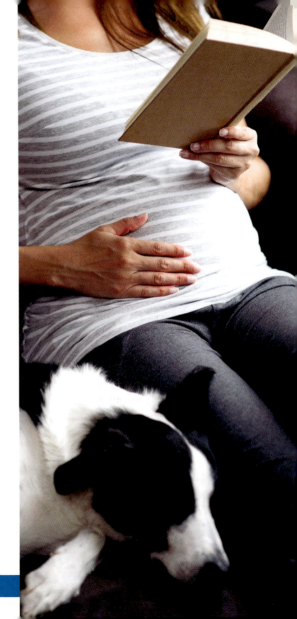

#56

All is calm

Tricks for being a baby whisperer:

- SOUND — For months in the womb, baby has been soothed by the low frequency sounds of blood whooshing and mom's rhythmic heartbeat. Simulate that environment by humming, saying "shh" or using a white noise machine. And your babe is probably the #1 fan of your singing, so entertain your captive audience often!
- MOVEMENT — Gentle movements such as swaying or mini squat-type dips may become your signature move.
- SUCKING — Sucking is a reflex and a need for babies. Feeding satisfies part of that need, but some babies need more and enjoy their own thumbs, fingers, an adult finger (clean!) or a pacifier. This need is strongest during the first few months and gradually tapers off.
- SNUGGLE — Think of how the fetal position is really a comfort zone at any age.

- RELAXING BREATHS — Try inhaling for a count of four, pause and hold breath for four counts, exhale for four counts, then hold breath out for four counts. Repeat. It'll help calm you — and baby may follow your lead.
- TOUCH — Baby will most likely love being massaged gently. Try long, downward, soothing strokes, or patting baby's back or bum. When you pick up and touch your baby, it can decrease both your and your baby's heart rates and blood pressures.
- FRESH AIR/FRESH PERSPECTIVE — Maybe stepping outside will be the ticket?
- WHITE NOISE — Standing near the sound of a fan, washer or dryer has been just the trick for many crying babies. There are apps and small machines for white noise, too.

TRY THESE THINGS EARLY — The sooner you respond to your baby's needs, the easier he or she will be soothed.

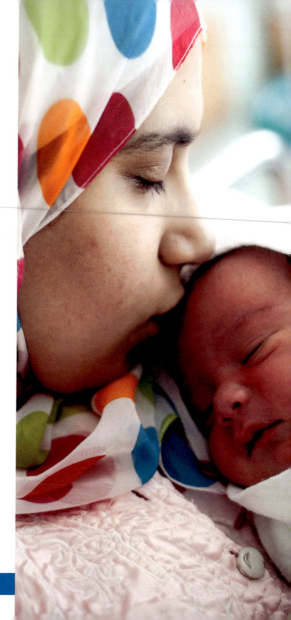

#57

About the back pages

The FLIP SIDE pages provide a bit more information to prepare you for birth and beyond. After all, knowledge is power. In addition to providing more medical info, these back pages include real-life birth stories and practical tips for once your newborn arrives. Some pages delve into what happens when labor doesn't go as planned and more intervention is needed. Others have space for you to jot notes and memories and attach an ultrasound photo to record your own personal journey.

Obstetricks aims to provide the most useful information for families looking ahead to a birth. Peruse the back pages for a more complete crash course, or refer back to the table of contents and jump to the pages that pique your interest most. We hope you will find these tips to be extremely helpful!

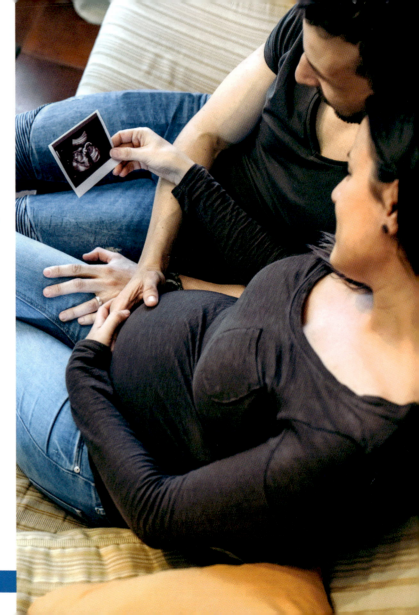